The Book of Exercise and Yoga for Those with Parkinson's Disease

Using Movement and Meditation to Manage Symptoms

(2nd Edition)

Copyright 2010 by Living Well Yoga and Fitness

All rights reserved. No part of this publication may be reproduced or transmitted in any form or by any means, electronic, mechanical, including photocopy, recording, or any other information storage and retrieval system, without the prior written permission of the publisher.

ISBN: 9781453641774

Published by:
Living Well Yoga and Fitness
www.lwyf.org

Acknowledgments

My sincere gratitude to my students living with Parkinson's disease who face each day's challenges with courage, grace and humor. Thank you for coming to class with your jokes and stories and for your compassion and friendship to each other and all who come to class. For just showing up and facing life's hurdles with humor, you are and will continue to be, an inspiration to us all.

Dedication

This book is dedicated to the more than six million people living with Parkinson's disease and their families. Proceeds from the sale of this book will be donated to help find a cure.

Note:

This book is provided as a helpful reference source only. It is not intended as a medical guide, or a guide for self-treatment. The suggestions herein are not intended to replace appropriate medical care. If you are concerned about your health or diagnosis, seek competent medical attention. This book offers techniques that may be helpful for those with Parkinson's disease. If you are living with another medical condition some of the suggestions in this book may be contraindicated for your condition. Check with your health care provider about the appropriateness of this program given your particular diagnosis.

Never exercise to the point of pain or strain. discontinue exercising immediately if you experience pain or pressure in the chest, dizziness, nausea, extreme muscle soreness, or a worsening of symptoms. If you should experience any of the above, consult your health care provider immediately.

Table of Contents

Acknowledgments and Dedication ……………………………..… 3

Forward……………………………………….....……………….6

Introduction
Making Exercise a Part of Your Day...…………………………..…..9

Chapter 1
Posture and Body Mechanics ..……………………………….....15

Chapter 2
Diaphragmatic Breathing and Warm Up Exercises ………....….…. ..47

Chapter 3
Aerobic Exercise ………… ……………………………….. ..77

Chapter 4
Strength Training…...…….... …………………………….......97

Chapter 5
Yoga and Tai Chi for Flexibility and Balance ..…………...................128

Chapter 6
Relaxation Techniques and Stress Management ..………....…....189

Appendix ..……………………………………………….......205
Workout Logs, Sample Routines

Resource Section ……………………………………….......227
Helpful websites

Forward

The word disease has been defined by Brian Langlois, religious science minister as meaning "without harmony, out of balance or ill at ease". People with Parkinson's disease often define their relationship with their environment in similar terms due to the multiple symptoms that they experience with this chronic disease. Advances in research have lead to medications that help to control the symptoms and restore a feeling of balance or harmony at least for brief periods of time during their day.

Exercise has been shown to benefit everyone at every age. Exercise produces natural endorphins that stimulate the body and restore balance and harmony. Yoga is an ancient science that helps to restore balance and harmony among the mind, body and spirit. The combination of physical exercise (asanas) and breathing exercise (pranayama) with meditation in yoga bring unity to the mind, body and spirit.

People with Parkinson's disease are slowly robbed of their ability to perform activities automatically. It becomes necessary to concentrate on each movement. The practice of yoga creates unity between mind and body, allowing intentional movement. Yoga is a non-competitive activity, emphasizing slow deliberate movements that enhance mindfulness and awareness. Although there are numerous books and videotapes available on the subject of yoga, almost none deal with the specific challenges of Parkinson's. Research indicates that people with Parkinson's disease who practice yoga regularly have improved flexibility, balance, posture and mood. The relaxation achieved through yoga has been shown to allow stretched muscles to maintain their elongation long after exercise has ended.

Parkinson's disease does affect muscle flexibility for most people with this chronic disease. Loss of flexibility leads to postural misalignment. Poor posture and body mechanics can lead to devastating falls. *The Book of Exercise and Yoga for Those with Parkinson's Disease* addresses posture and body mechanics in a practical manner, demonstrating how activities of daily living can be performed safely. I have found that the first chapter of this book is a vital resource for people with Parkinson's disease as well as other professionals. Each activity is demonstrated as well as explained, making it a valuable guide to help people with Parkinson's follow the step by step instructions for safely performing tasks that are no longer automatic.

Postural problems are related to loss of flexibility as well as strength. Stronger muscles pull a body into misalignment. Exercises that strengthen the weaker muscles will help to achieve balance and prevent deformity. Lori Newell does a wonderful job of providing pictures of the muscles being strengthened as well as options for performing the activity in both sitting and standing. Having the option of exercising in both sitting and standing allows the person with this chronic disease to exercise even on those days when their symptoms are not well controlled with their medications.

It has been said that 'knowledge is power'. There are many misconceptions about yoga and people with Parkinson's disease and their caregivers often feel that yoga is too difficult or too demanding. In actuality, for those with Parkinson's, yoga is just what the doctor ordered. Living with Parkinson's Disease means taking time each day to take care of yourself. Yoga can play an integral part in helping you maintain a healthy lifestyle and quality of life. People with Parkinson's disease can regain a feeling of control by knowing how to modify their exercise regime to accommodate fluctuations of symptoms and by understanding how the mind, body and spirit are interconnected.

The Book of Exercise and Yoga for Those with Parkinson's Disease, includes information on the coordination of the body systems to achieve balance and harmony on many levels. The information on the 'stress response' is one example of the complexity of how a loss of harmony or balance of systems can lead to other chronic illnesses. Opening the mind to yoga as a means of healing and promoting physical, emotional and spiritual balance will do much to ensure that people with Parkinson's disease maintain quality of life. This book should be a constant companion and reference for all those who suffer from this chronic disease as well as for their caregivers, both family and professional.

Jeanne Csuy, PT, GCS, MS Outreach Coordinator for the Lee Parkinson's Outreach Center in Fort Myers, Florida

This book is a detailed, insightful resource for people with or without Parkinson's disease who are interested in developing an exercise routine. The diagrams and written instructions are broken into various levels of physical ability and are surrounded with many tips for making life easier.

Endorsed by Ann Zylstra PT
Booth Gardner Parkinson's Center
Kirkland WA

This book is full of practical exercises tailored specifically to the needs of people with Parkinson disease. As evidence of the benefits of exercise on mind and body grows yearly this is a hopeful, promising and user friendly resource for people with Parkinson and their caregivers. In addition to simple stretching exercises suggestions for incorporating exercise into daily life are offered. An important contribution and a great tool for people living well with Parkinson disease!

Laura S. Boylan, MD
Medical Director Bellevue Hospital
Parkinson and Movement Disorders Center
New York City, NY

Introduction

Using Movement and Meditation To Manage the Symptoms of Parkinson's Disease

"Life affords no higher pleasure than that of surmounting difficulties, passing from one step of success to another, forming new wishes, and seeing them gratified. He that labors in any great or laudable undertaking has his fatigues first supported by hope, and afterwards rewarded by joy...To strive with difficulties, and to conquer them, is the highest human felicity."
-Samuel Johnson

    This book provides an outline of the exercise and yoga program I teach for those with Parkinson's Disease. Many of my students would often miss classes due to doctor or physical therapy appointments and during the winter months classes would often be canceled due to the weather. My students and their caregivers often asked me for written information so they could exercise at home when they could not make it to class. My students then began to share this book with others affected by PD. As I continued to receive feedback on how helpful this program is in managing the symptoms of PD I decided to update the information and publish this book so others can hopefully benefit from the information. While it is always best to exercise with a knowledgeable instructor to prevent injury and ensure that you are exercising correctly, this book can be used as a supplement on days you can not get to class. I hope you find the information helpful and remember to always work at your own pace.

What is Parkinson's Disease

    Parkinson's disease is a neurological disorder first described in 1817 by Dr. James Parkinson. It is characterized by tremor or shaking of the limbs, slower movements, rigidity or stiffness especially in the trunk of the body, and loss of balance. Everyday activities may become more difficult to perform, and the symptoms may be worse on one side then the other. Other changes can include small cramped handwriting, absence of facial expression, scuffing of feet when walking, speech becoming softer and more difficult for others to hear, depression, and a forward stooping posture. These changes in posture and gait can oftentimes increase your tendency to fall. The types of symptoms present and the rate at which this disease progresses, can vary greatly from person to person.
    Parkinson's disease results when nerve cells in the substantia nigra area of the brain die or become impaired. As these dopamine-producing cells become damaged, the symptoms of Parkinson's disease appear. Dopamine is a neurotransmitter involved in coordinating smooth and

balanced muscle movement. As these cells are impaired and less dopamine is available, nerve cells fire out of control causing tremors, or difficulty initiating movement. Parkinson's disease is often difficult to diagnose because there are no specific x-rays or blood tests that can help to determine its presence. It can be diagnosed only through observation and thorough examination.

Current estimates by the National Parkinson's Foundation indicate that approximately six million people worldwide have Parkinson's disease, and another 60,000 new cases are diagnosed each year. It affects both men and women equally and does not appear to affect a particular social, ethnic, economic, or geographical group. The average age of onset is in the early sixties, although approximately ten percent of those diagnosed experience onset at age forty or younger.

How Exercise and Yoga Can Help

Since there is currently no cure for the disease, treatment is aimed at managing the symptoms, working to maintain independent function, and as much as possible reducing disability from the disease. Treatment can include medication, surgery, and healthy lifestyle habits, including daily exercise. Daily exercise and movement are essential to help curb the stiffness and rigidity that occurs, to help lift mood, and to provide opportunities to connect with others. While exercise cannot cure the disease, an appropriate exercise routine may help to slow the progression of the condition, allowing you to minimize its effects. Participating in daily exercise can improve your lung capacity, muscle strength, balance, gait, the ability to initiate movement, and flexibility.

The program in this book is an invitation to explore various types of movement and meditation as ways to manage the symptoms of Parkinson's disease. The following chapters outline the program I have been teaching to my students with Parkinson's. Each chapter explains and illustrates various types of activity. You are not expected to do every exercise or movement in this book every day. Each chapter will examine different components of an exercise regimen, and explain how to develop an appropriate exercise routine. The resource section includes sample workout logs and routines to help you create the program that best fits your needs.

Exercise alone can not cure this terrible disease, but in the long run it can help lift your spirits, improve everyday functioning, and help you to feel less victimized by your condition. I hope you find this program helpful. Please know that you are in my thoughts and my heart as you continue on your journey.

Peggy's Story:

Before I was diagnosed with Parkinson's disease, I never met an exercise I liked! As a travel writer, I enjoyed penning articles about my disdain for the athletic life. "A NON-ATHLETE'S FEAT, my most popular article ever, boasted of clever ways I devised to get out of participating in sporting events. As for hiking, backpacking and skiing, I can truthfully say, that like Woody Allen, I was at TWO WITH NATURE. When I was talked into a camping trip by two of my naturalist friends, I was such a novice I took an Electric Blanket -- This camping faux pas ended up as a headline (Don't bring an electric blanket on a Camping Trip) for a travel article I wrote for The San Francisco Examiner & Chronicle.

What a difference a disease makes!! Before exercising was optional, and I opted out of it. Now exercising isn't a choice; it's a given. It's my job. Because Parkinson's disease is a movement disorder, movement is a good way to combat it. Exercise is now considered by most authorities to be the new medicine for people with Parkinson's disease. Lucky for you there's a great new book for people with PD. Lori Newell's tome, *The Book of Exercise and Yoga for Those with Parkinson's Disease,* is a superb compilation and I highly recommend it for people with Parkinson's, their families and friends.

When I was first diagnosed with PD almost seven years ago, I knew I should exercise, but I had no idea what type of exercise to do. When I was writing an article about Parkinson's and Yoga for Yoga Journal a few years later, I discovered, Newell's book, the very book I wished I had had from the get-go.

The exercises are well explained, easy to do and not intimidating, and they feel good. The Alternate Straight Leg Kick is the perfect solution for my Parkinson-caused leg cramps. To reduce the stiffness in my left arm, I like the Chest Stretch which has the added benefit of correcting posture, always a problem for people with PD. Newell has some great advice on how to combat "freezing" (what I call doing my imitation of the Tin Man in The Wizard of Oz and can hardly move). My favorite tip is singing or humming an easy song that you know well so you create a rhythm for your body to follow.

As a Stress A+ personality type, I was fascinated by the section of the book explaining how harmful stress can be to a person (like me) with PD. I was horrified to learn stress can even speed up your disease. I was delighted to see the next section was on meditation. I tried a few meditation exercises and found them to be very relaxing.

As an author researching and writing a book about my Parkinson's journey, I found Newell's book helpful in all regards. She is a treasure trove of information and I learned an enormous amount to help with my book and articles and more importantly about how to deal with my own PD symptoms. This is a book everyone with Parkinson's should have in their library.
- Peggy van Hulsteyn

Making Exercise a Part of Your Day

The benefits of regular exercise have been well documented. Hardly a day goes by when we are not reminded of its importance through news broadcasts, newspapers, and magazine articles. Regular exercise combined with other healthy lifestyle choices can help one to manage weight, reduce blood pressure, cholesterol levels, and stress. It can also aid in the prevention and management of such conditions as diabetes, heart disease, cancer, arthritis, and osteoporosis. While exercise can help to moderate many conditions, it is especially crucial for those who are living with a chronic disease. In the case of Parkinson's disease, the body is being affected by a progressive condition which can cause a loss of mobility. The ability to do everyday activities becomes more challenging as joints lose range of motion, muscles become weaker, balance is compromised, and breathing capacity is more limited.

Daily activities such as eating, dressing, bathing, sleeping, toileting or walking can become more difficult for those with Parkinson's disease. Typical symptoms of Parkinson's disease such as tremor, stiffness, slow movement, and balance problems may worsen over time, and can make it more difficult to do such things as getting in and out of a car, standing up from a chair, or walking.

Addressing these symptoms with regular exercise may help as one maintains or even gains more mobility. A complete exercise program should consist of three components, aerobic or cardiovascular exercise, strength training exercise, and stretching exercises. Regular aerobic exercise helps make the heart stronger and increases lung capacity. Strength training exercises help to improve muscular strength and stability. Stretching exercises help maintain joint range of motion and flexibility. The following chapters will explore these three components and discuss in detail how they can help.

Fitting exercise into your daily routine can be challenging especially when you are also dealing with a chronic disease. There are some steps you can take to make this easier:

1) *Schedule Your Exercise Session On Your Calender*
Schedule your exercise session into your day as you would a doctor's appointment or a meeting with a friend, and do not break your appointment unless it is absolutely necessary. Postponing your designated time can become a habit too easy to maintain. This could result in neglecting exercise altogether. Exercise is an important component to your overall health. Your exercise schedule should be given a priority as important as a medical appointment.

2) *Pick a Time of Day When You Feel Your Best*
Schedule your exercise routine for a time of day that works best for you. For those with Parkinson's disease, this means finding a time when your medications are working and you feel your strongest. If you know that your medication wears off by late afternoon, make sure you schedule your session earlier in the day.

3) *Exercise with Someone*
Exercising with a partner or friend is more enjoyable then going at it alone. It keeps you motivated and on track. Making an agreement to do this is a great way to help you stick to your routine. Even if you do not feel like exercising you may not want to let your partner down.

4) *Do What You Can in the Time You Have*
If you have time to do only part of your usual routine, do what you can. Do not skip your exercise session just because you have time for only part of it. Because unavoidable situations may occur to disrupt your routine, you may be tempted to skip it, a practice that too easily leads to breaking your exercise habit altogether. Missing one exercise session may tempt you to miss the next day, and before long you may stop exercising altogether. By doing what you can in the time allowed helps you to maintain a rhythm of regular exercise.

5) *If You Fall Off Track, Start Again the Very Next Day*
Should you fall off track, do not be too hard on yourself. Everyone experiences periods of slipping back into old habits and routines. The important thing is that you recognize this pattern and return quickly to healthier habits and lifestyle choices. There will be times when sticking to your routine seems easy, and other times when it seems like a hard chore. If you do fall off track there is a temptation to say "I'll start again next week, or next month..." This just takes you out of your routine for an even longer period of time. If you miss your session on Monday, get right back to it on Tuesday. There is no reason to wait and put it off. The longer you can stick with your regular routine the easier it will be to get back on track, if and when you falter.

6) *Have a List of Why Exercise is Important and Look at it Frequently*
Make a reasonable and realistic list of the reasons why you decided to start exercising and go back to it frequently. It might include such things as being able to climb stairs, putting your shoes on more easily, or reducing the risk of a fall. Periodically remind yourself how staying with an exercise regimen can help improve the quality of your life, and your ability to remain independent.

7) *Keep Records of Your Accomplishments and Efforts*
Keep progress reports or workout logs of your exercise sessions. There is nothing more motivating then seeing results. Benefits can appear as early as four to eight weeks. Within this time period you may notice that some everyday activities have become easier. If you look back at your workout log you may be surprised at how many more repetitions of each exercise you can now complete, or how much more aerobic activity you can tolerate.

How to Use This Book

The most important thing is to exercise on a regular basis! This book covers a wide variety of techniques to get you moving and help you to manage your symptoms. Each chapter will explain why the different techniques are important and how they affect your body and your symptoms. You do not need to do every exercise in this book every day. I would suggest briefly reading through each chapter first to get an idea of the different techniques and how to incorporate them into your routine. At the end of the book there is an appendix with sample routines and workout logs to help you design the program that works best for you. After reading through the book then go back and start to try some of the exercises. Remember to start gradually and never do more then feels right. As your body becomes stronger and more flexible slowly add on additional exercises.

Continue to explore the suggestions and techniques written here and look into other books, videos and programs as well. Try various approaches. Then work to find the best solution for your situation. Parkinson's disease affects each person differently. You are the best judge of what feels right for your body. Through experimentation you will find the routine that suits your needs and helps you to accomplish your goals.

Chapter One

Posture and Body Mechanics

"Success is that peace of mind that comes from knowing you've done everything in your power to become the very best you're capable of becoming."
- John Wooden

    While adhering to a regular exercise routine can help you manage the symptoms of many conditions, it is equally important to be mindful of how you use your body during everyday activities. If your goal is to improve posture, you can perform the exercises that will help you to reach that goal. However, if you then spend the rest of your day sitting incorrectly, or lifting objects improperly, you will undo all of the benefits of your exercise session. Also, remember that incorrect posture and body mechanics can increase your chances of a fall. This chapter covers some of the basics of good posture and body mechanics.

    First, let us examine good posture. Having Parkinson's disease can cause postural changes in the body such as a forward head position, rounding of the shoulders and upper back, and a forward trunk position with increased bending at the hips and knees. Some common activities during which we may use incorrect posture include sitting in general, watching TV, working at a computer, driving and riding in a car, looking downward while reading, household chores, and yard work.

    The remainder of this chapter will explore common everyday activities and chores and suggest ways of doing them that are safer and easier on the joints. By taking the time to take care of your body you will reduce your risk for a fall and/or other injury so you can remain active and independent.

The following are some basic body mechanics principles to help correct posture, make everyday activities easier, and reduce the risk of falls.

- Bend or hinge at the hips, not the waist.
- When bending, squat. Knees should be bent, back should be straight.
- You are more steady with the feet wider apart and staggered. You are less steady with the feet closer together and parallel to each other.
- If lifting or bending compromises your balance, place your feet about hip width apart with one foot in front of the other for more stability.
- It is easier and more safe to push. It is harder and less safe to pull.
- Carry objects close to your body.
- When pushing or moving objects, use your body weight and momentum to push. Do not rely solely on arm strength.
- Lift with your legs, not your back.
- Always test the weight of the object before you try to lift it.
- Reorganize your house so that items you commonly use are within easy reach, preferably at a level between your knees and shoulders.
- Do not twist when lifting or pushing.
- When sweeping, vacuuming, shoveling, raking, etc., always face your work and move with it. Your nose, knees and toes should all be facing in the same direction.
- When performing the above mentioned activities, use a rocking motion, by transferring your weight from one leg to the other as you move. This allows your leg muscles to help with the work.

Avoiding Falls

Many accidents happen in the kitchen and bathroom. Falls can happen while walking around, rising from a sitting position, and stepping out of the shower. The following are some tips for preventing falls.

- Be aware of the medications you take and their side effects. Some can increase the risk of falls.
- Try to avoid reaching out to furniture or handrails while walking.
Stooping forward and reaching ahead of you can bring you out of balance and cause a fall.
- Be aware of uneven surfaces in rooms.
- Immediately wipe up any spilled liquids.
- Do not use scatter rugs that might slide on the floor. Secure them with skid-proof backing or securely tack them down. Worn or frayed rugs can cause tripping.
- If you need to use a step stool, make sure it is sturdy and secure.
- Always wear non-skid socks or slippers instead of regular socks.
- When rising from a lying down or a seated position, move slowly to avoid becoming dizzy.
- Make sure you have adequate lighting throughout the house. Use night lights at night.
- Keep all floors clear of clutter.
- Before starting any activity, think it through! Make sure you place everything you need in an easy-to-get-to spot.
- Make a plan for getting help should you fall or become hurt.
- Try to locate phones throughout the house especially in areas such as the bathroom and kitchen where most accidents happen. As much as possible use cordless or cell phones you can carry with you. Place the phones at a level you can reach should you be unable to get up off the floor.
- If you live alone, check in with someone on a regular basis in the event that you need help and are unable to get to a phone.
- Wear a medical alert bracelet or necklace if you fall frequently. With the push of a button, medical help will arrive quickly.

Hip Hinge

Before examining specific activities we will learn about a movement called the hip hinge. This involves reaching the buttocks back as if you were going to sit in a chair, bending at the knees, keeping a natural arch in the low back and coming forward by bending at the hips instead of the waist.

This movement should be used when:

- Getting up and down from a chair
- Getting in and out of a car
- Lifting items off the floor or out of lower cabinets
- Shoveling, vacuuming, and cleaning
- Taking items in and out of an oven, washer, or dryer
- Anytime you need to stoop but cannot get down on one knee

When hip hinging bend at your hips instead of your waist. The shoulders come forward, the back stays straight, head up, and as you bend your knees reach your hips back as if you were about to sit in a chair.

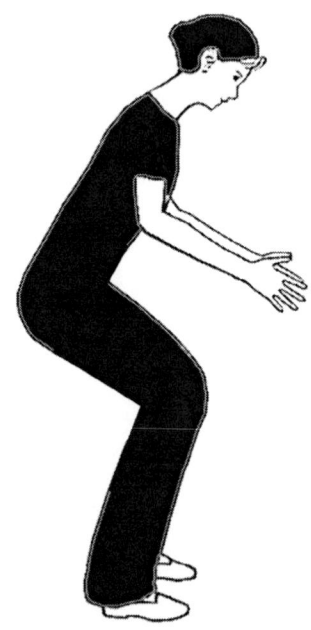

Correct Sitting

As discussed earlier in this book to best manage your symptoms it is important to be mindful of how you use your body during everyday activities. Most of us spend a large portion of the day sitting. Since Parkinson's Disease can cause a rounding of the shoulders and upper back learning to sit correctly throughout the day can play a large role in helping to correct your posture.

Some things to keep in mind include:

- Avoid recliners. They promote rounding of the neck, shoulders and head, and tightness in the hips. Avoid low, soft couches and chairs that make rising difficult. Instead choose a chair of average height with firm, smooth cushions and sturdy armrests.
- The height of the chair should allow for your hips and knees to be level with one another, or for the hips to be slightly higher than the knees.
- When sitting up straight do not tilt the head back. Keep your chin parallel to the floor.
- Avoid crossing your legs as this will increase tightness in the hips.
- Both your computer screen and TV should be at eye level to minimize neck strain.
- While reading, use a book stand or rest your elbows on a pillow or table.
- A good general rule is to *change your posture every fifteen to twenty minutes*. At this point, get up and move around. Sitting for longer periods leads to stiffness and poor circulation, both of which can trigger a fall when you try to stand.
- Chairs should have a stable base. Swivel or rocking chairs are not a good choice because they can trigger loss of balance.
- To make it easier to stand up from a lower chair, raise the seat height by adding an extra cushion. Electric lift chairs and lift cushions can be helpful for people who have trouble getting out of chairs.

Correct Sitting Posture

Use the guidelines below to check that you are sitting correctly.

- Keep your ears over your shoulders and your shoulders over your hips. Do not round the back or slouch in the chair
- Keep your back straight but not rigid, allowing for the natural curve to remain in the low back.
- Your feet should be flat on the floor. If your feet do not reach, place a book or stool underneath them
- Sit up straight by pushing the crown of the head to the ceiling, but keep your chin parallel to the floor. Do not tilt the head back.
- Your abdominal muscles should be lightly tucked in and your shoulders down and relaxed and away from your ears.

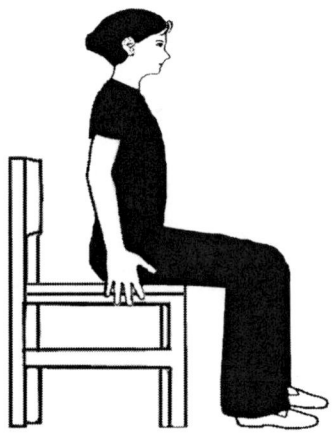

As much as you can throughout the day try to sit towards the front of the chair. This helps to avoid slouching and it will strengthen the abdominal and back muscles by making them work to hold you up. Do not sit this way for too long at first. Try sitting this way for brief periods throughout the day, (when working at the computer and at the dinner table). Slowly increase the time you sit this way each day. When you need to sit back, slide the buttocks all the way back in the chair in order to keep the ears over the shoulders and the shoulders over hips. Avoid just leaning back and slouching in the chair.

Getting In and Out of a Chair

Falls often happen when moving from sitting to standing or standing to sitting. Protect your body and back by carefully lowering yourself in and lifting yourself out of chairs.

Steps to Transition from Sitting to Standing

1. Bring your hips forward to the very edge of the chair (or couch) because it is more difficult to get up if you are sitting at the back of the chair.
2. Feet should be approximately shoulder-width apart or wider to provide a good base of support.
3. Position the feet either parallel to each other or place your stronger leg slightly back.

        Feet parallel.   One leg slightly back.

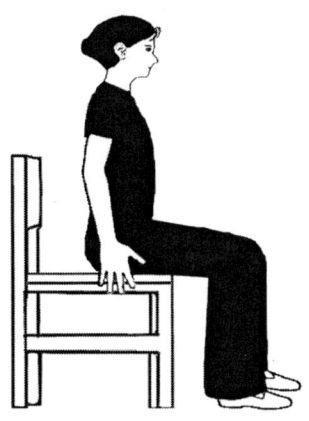 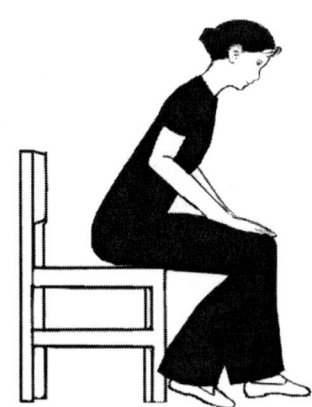

4. Lean forward at the hips until your head is positioned nose over knees and toes.

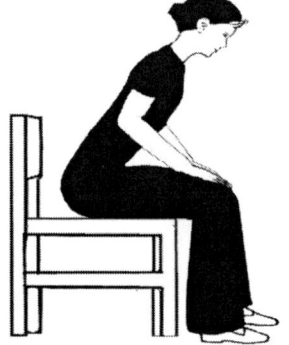

21

5. Continue to lean forward, bringing the nose over the toes to come up to standing. Let your legs do most of the work. Try to push off of your thighs to get up. Your leg muscles are much larger and stronger than those in your arms. If your legs are not strong enough to lift you up, you can push off the seat or arms of the chair, but avoid relying on arm strength alone to lift yourself up.

Keep your back straight and look slightly down and ahead of you.

Getting up pushing off of your thighs

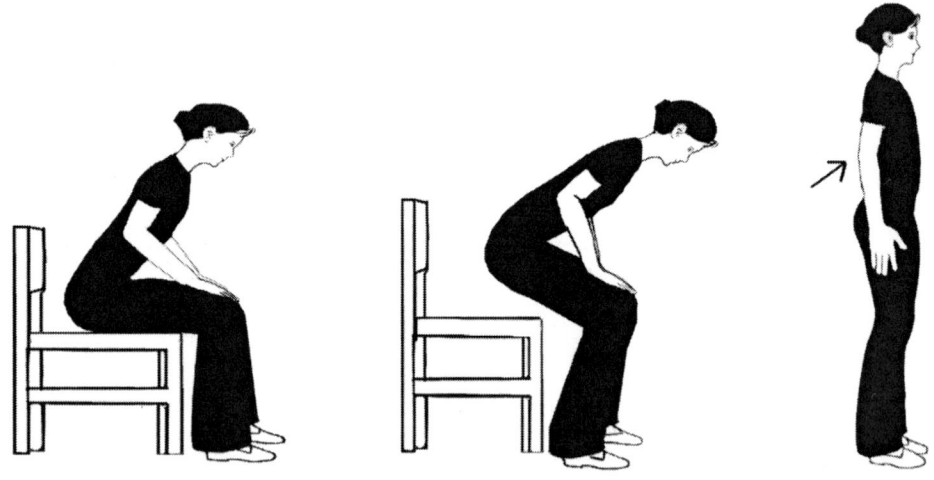

Getting up pushing off of the seat of the chair

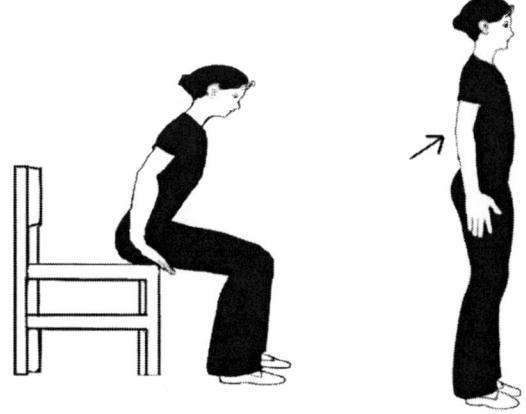

Getting up pushing off of the arms of a chair

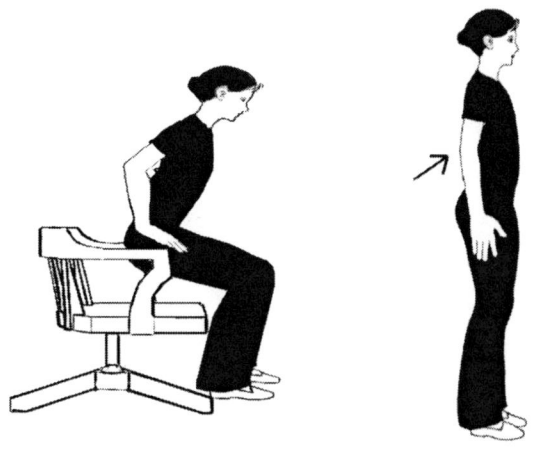

Steps to Transition from Standing to Sitting

Take large rather then short shuffling steps as you approach the chair.

1. Position yourself so the chair is centered directly behind you. You should feel the chair against the back of your legs before sitting.
2. Reach back for the seat or armrests as you "hip hinge" forward. Think nose over knees and toes.
3. Keep your back straight, head up and eyes forward. Do not reach for the chair before you turn to sit; you might lose your balance or fall.
4. Use your leg strength to lower your body *slowly and gently* to the edge of the chair. Then slide back. If your legs are not strong enough to lower yourself to the chair, use your arms to help control your descent.
  Avoid crashing down into a chair. Crashing down into a chair can cause injury to the back and oftentimes triggers a fall.

Sitting down using the seat of the chair

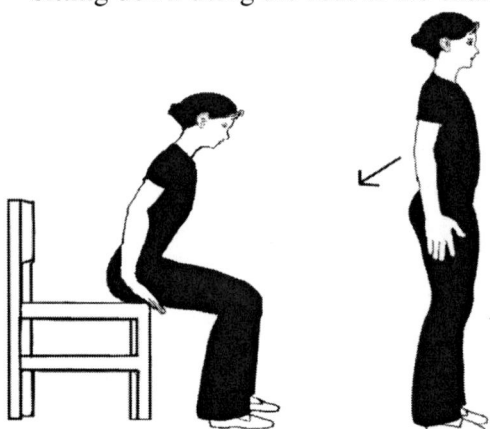

Sitting down using the arms of a chair

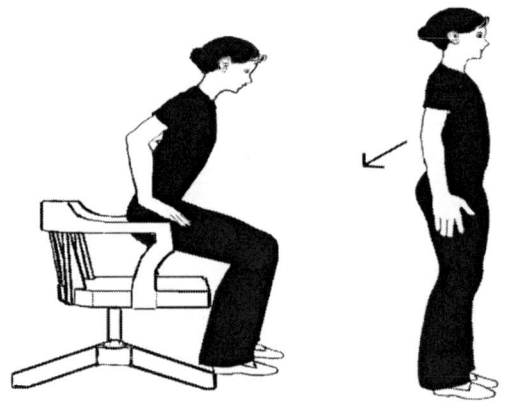

Steps To Safely Get In and Out of a Car

Always avoid stepping from a curb into a car, or from a car onto a curb. Remember always; from ground level to car, from car to ground level.

To get into a car

Always avoid getting into a car sideways.
1. Approach the car seat the same way you would a chair. Turn so your back is to the seat with your buttocks leading the way.
2. Reach back for the seat or dashboard and slowly lower yourself onto the seat. Land so you are sitting at the edge of the seat. Do not hold on to the door which can move and trigger a fall.
3. With one hand hold onto the seat inside the car. With the other hand lift one leg at a time into the car. Then you can turn your body on the seat to face forward.
4. Place a plastic bag on cloth seats to make turning easier.

To get out of a car

Always avoid getting out of a car sideways.
1. Hold onto the dashboard with one hand. With the other hand, lift one leg at a time out of the car.
2. Then you can turn your body on the seat to face out.
3. You should be sitting in the car with both of your legs out of the car and feet flat on the ground.
4. Then, move the buttocks forward to the edge of the car seat and lean forward (hip hinge) while pushing up from the seat or dashboard. Do not pull up on the car door, which can move and trigger a fall.

Standing Correctly

Since having Parkinson's disease can cause tightness in the chest it is common for those with PD to stand with a rounded back and shoulders. This puts a strain on the low back and can lead to chronic back pain, In addition it brings your weight forward and out of balance which can trigger a fall. If you go on for years with poor posture, eventually your muscles will become accustomed to this and you may no longer feel any discomfort or even be aware of when you are standing incorrectly. Since this change in posture is musculature it can be corrected. Throughout the day check your posture and remind yourself to stand up straight. With constant practice the muscles will be retrained. Eventually it will start to feel incorrect when you are leaning forward and better posture will feel more comfortable.

Correct Standing Tips

- Keep your chin parallel to the floor.
- Maintain a broad base of support by keeping your feet shoulder width apart or wider.
- Abdominal muscles should be in, shoulders back and down, head and chest up, and knees slightly bent, but never locked.
- An easy way to help you stand straight is to think about lifting the top of your head to the ceiling. Do not lift your chin, your chin stays parallel with the floor. As you focus on lifting the top of the head up, you may feel yourself standing taller as your abdominal and waist muscles tighten.

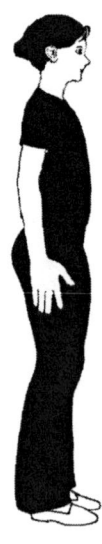

Walking Correctly

Walking smoothly and with good balance can be challenging for those with Parkinson's Disease. There is a tendency to take short, quick shuffling steps on the toes. This type of walking is often the cause of falls. Falls occur since you are scuffing the toes which can catch on carpeting or rough surfaces causing you to trip and fall. It is better to take longer, slower strides which gives your body a chance to balance itself. It is also important to focus on picking the feet up, flexing the foot and landing with the heel down and the toes lifted. In addition, the faster you walk the more momentum you create. If you start to lose your balance it will be harder to stop a fall then if you are taking slower and longer strides and putting the heel down first.

Correct Walking Tips

- Do not look straight down while walking, look ahead and slightly down.
- Look down with your eyes, not your head.
- Keep your hands free. Carry light loads in small body packs. For those with PD trying to carry items and walk at the same time may be more than the brain can process, which can lead to freezing. Keeping the hands free so they can swing as you walk, may help to prevent freezing.
- If balance or strength is affecting your ability to walk, use a mobility aid (cane, walker or walking stick) adjusted to the proper height.
- When stepping out flex your front foot, letting your heel strike first.
- Landing with the heel first and toes up forces you to pick up your feet, lessening the risk of tripping and falling.
- When you walk, swing your arms. A common characteristic of those with Parkinson's is walking with stiff arms. Try to swing the arm that is opposite to the forward foot. This helps you maintain balance, reduces the risk of falls, and provides momentum.
- Take long strides when you walk. Step out at least one foot's width distance with each step.

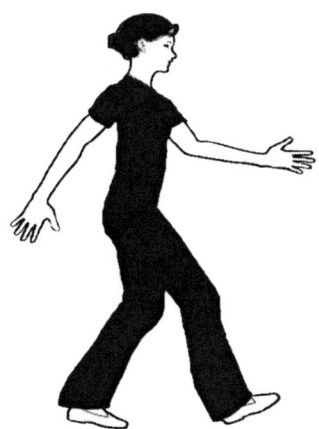

Lying Down and Getting In and Out of Bed

It is common for those with Parkinson's disease to have trouble turning over and with getting in and out of bed. Lying on your back with a soft pillow under the knees, or on your side with a soft pillow between the knees are the best postures for sleeping. It is also good to avoid using too many pillows, or too thin of a pillow under the head. Avoid sleeping in a chair. When napping lie down so that the head and neck are supported.

Tips for rolling or turning over in bed
- A satin sheet or piece of satin material placed on the bed can make it easier to turn over.
- Heavy weight blankets and flannel sheets can make turning over more difficult.
- To turn bend your knees and put your feet flat on the bed. Let your knees to fall to one side as you begin to roll. Turn your head in the direction you are rolling and reach the top arm across the body.
- A straight back chair anchored at the side of the bed or a bed rail can help you roll more easily.

Tips for scooting over in bed
- Bend your knees placing the feet flat on the bed.
- Push into the bed with both feet and hands to lift the hips up. Next shift the hips in the direction you wish to move. Then reposition your feet in the direction your hips moved.

Helpful bedroom aids

- A helping handle or bed rail that attaches between the mattress and box spring provides assistance with rolling, and support for pushing yourself to an upright position. An inexpensive alternative to a bed rail is a straight-back chair securely laced to the bed frame.
- An adjustable blanket support keeps the blanket off your feet, making it easier to move.
- A motion-activated night light detects movement and automatically switches on if you have to get up in the middle of the night.
- Electric beds make it easy to elevate your head and upper body, making breathing easier.

Steps For Safely Getting Into Bed

1. Back up to the bed just as you would to a chair; make sure you can feel the mattress behind both legs before you sit. Reach back for the bed with your hands.
2. Slowly lower yourself onto the edge of the bed using your leg muscles to control your descent. Use the hip hinge motion (pg.18).

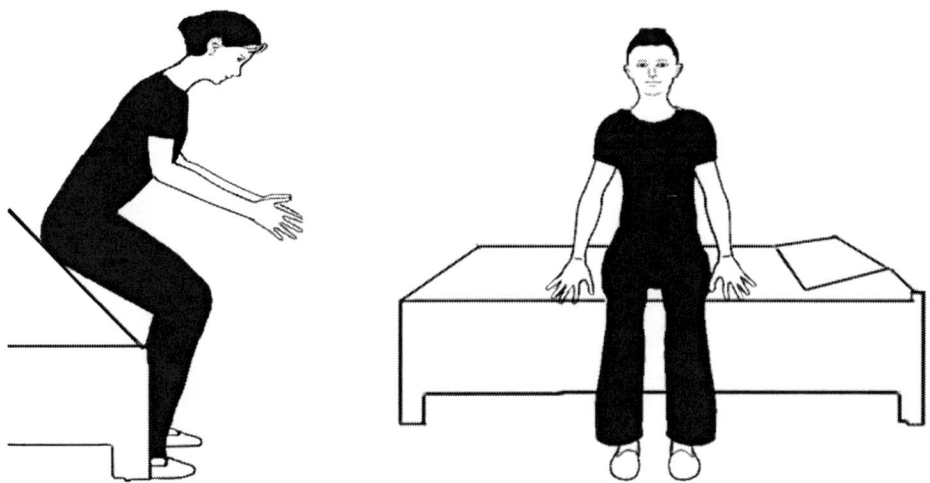

3. As your trunk goes down, bring the legs up (like a seesaw motion).

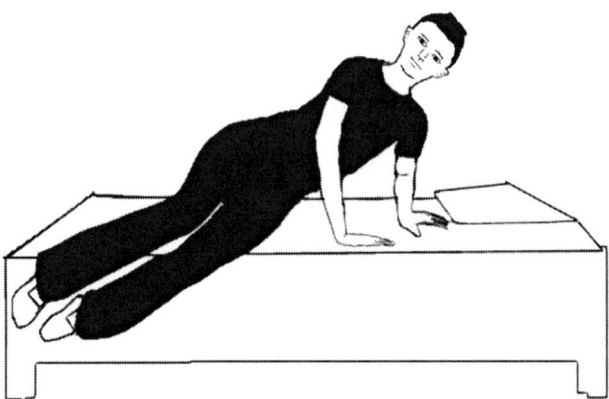

4. Use your arms to lower yourself onto your side.

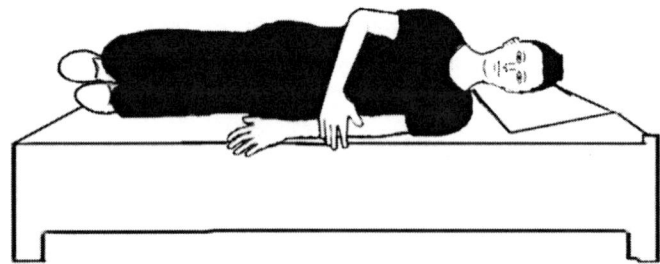

5. From here you can roll onto your back.

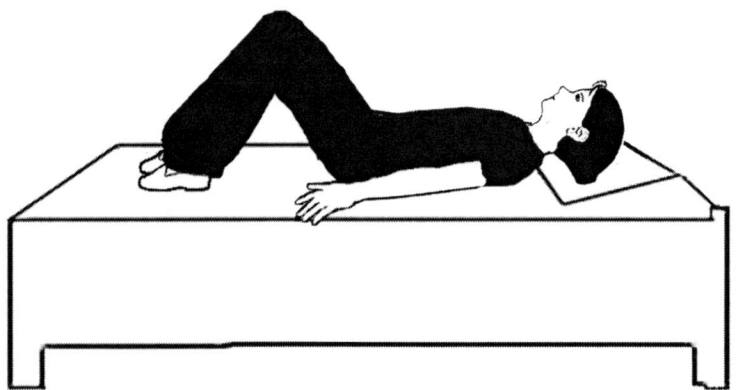

Steps For Safely Getting Out of Bed

1. Bend the knees up and place your feet flat on the bed. Reach across with the top arm. Turn your head and look in the direction you are rolling. Let the knees fall to the side so the body moves as a unit.

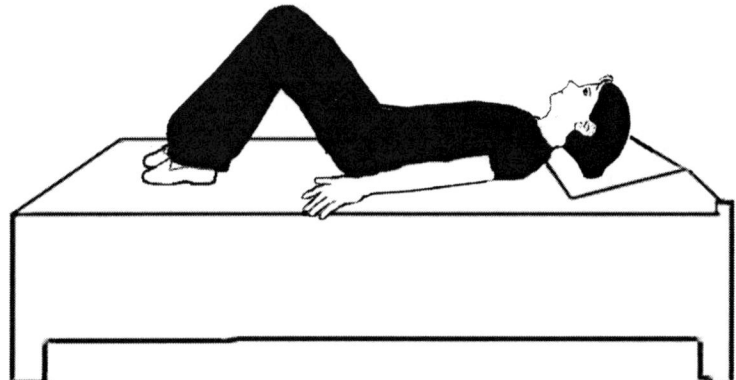

2. Roll all the way onto your side toward the edge of the bed. Push with your arms to lift the body up.

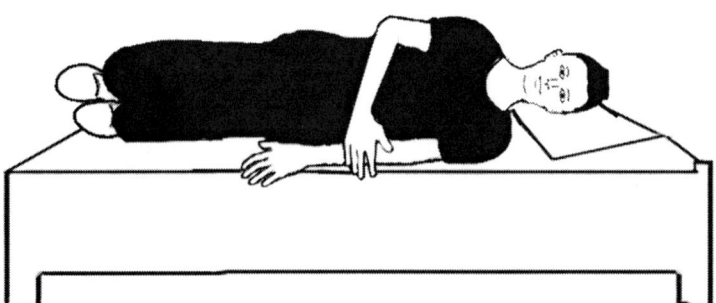

3. As your body comes up, let the legs slide off the side of the bed.

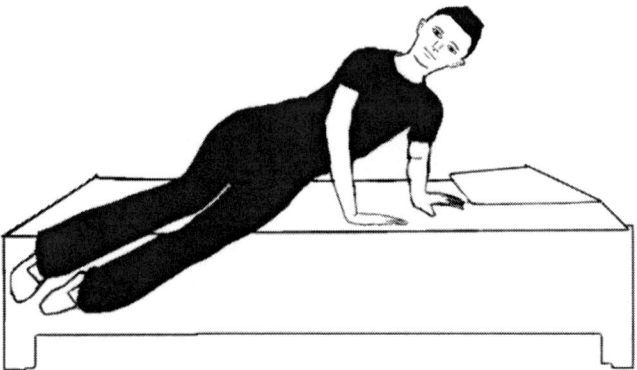

4. Lower feet towards the floor as you push with your arms into a sitting position. Slide to the edge of the bed, place the feet flat on the floor and use your legs to come to standing. Use the hip hinge motion (pg. 18).

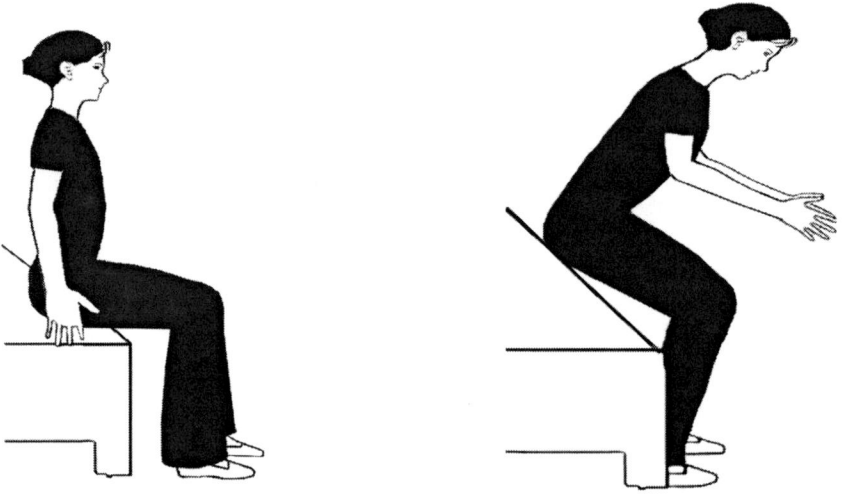

Avoid coming to a sitting position directly from your back. This strains the back muscles and is a more difficult way to get up. It is much safer to roll to your side before coming to a seated position.

Bathing, Grooming and Toileting

One of the most common places falls happen in the home is the bathroom. To help keep yourself safe try these tips.

Bathing Tips

- Shower stalls are much easier and safer to get into and out of than bathtubs so they are a better choice for bathing. If you decide to use a bathtub, try a tub transfer bench to help you get in and out more easily. Shower chairs are a good choice because they allow you to sit down while you shower. Putting on a terry robe after bathing also makes drying easier.
- There should be at least two grab bars near all tubs and shower stalls so you can hold on when getting in and out.
- Grab bars should always be professionally installed.
- A towel bar, soap dish, or faucet should never be used as a handrail. They are not secure enough to hold your body weight.
- When using a tub transfer bench or shower chair while showering, try a hand-held shower head. You can hold the shower head while you sit and then direct the water away from you to adjust the temperature safely.
- Have a non-skid rubber bath mat in all tubs and shower stalls.
- Make sure there is rubber backing on all bath rugs.
- Be careful when using bar soap. It is slippery, hard to hold, and can make the tub slippery if dropped. Pump soap containers or soap-on-a-rope are better choices.
- A night light should be kept on in the bathroom for times when you have to get up in the middle of the night.
- Whenever bathing alone, make sure you have a cordless or cell phone with you in case you fall and need help. Make sure you put the phone in a place you can easily reach from the floor, should you fall.

Grooming Tips

The rigidity and tremor common in Parkinson's disease can make it hard to handle toothbrushes, razors and hairdryers. Try the following ideas to make it easier.

- Sit down when brushing your teeth, shaving, and combing or drying your hair. Sitting down reduces the risk of falling and it helps you to conserve energy. A shower or commode chair is a good idea if standing and balancing is difficult. When using a chair try leaving the doors underneath the sink open to make room for your knees.
- You can also try a hands-free hairdryer mounted on a vanity so you do not have to use arm strength to hold the dryer.

Helpful bathing, grooming and toileting aids:

- A tub transfer bench or shower chair with a back adds extra safety for those who tire easily.
- An extra-long hand-held shower spray allows you to shower while seated on a bath chair in the tub.
- Commode frames or raised toilet seats make it easier to sit down and get up from the toilet.
- Lever faucet adapters ease grasping and turning.
- A long-handled sponge or brush helps people with limited range of motion reach the back and legs.

Remember to think about your body mechanics during all activities. For example, when brushing your teeth, try to avoid rounding the back when using the sink. Keep the back straight and bend the knees instead.

Correct
Knees bent, back straight.

Incorrect
Knees locked, back
and shoulders rounded.

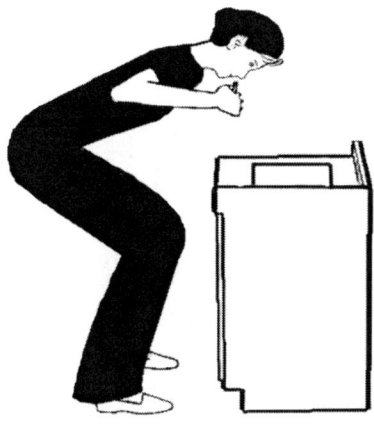 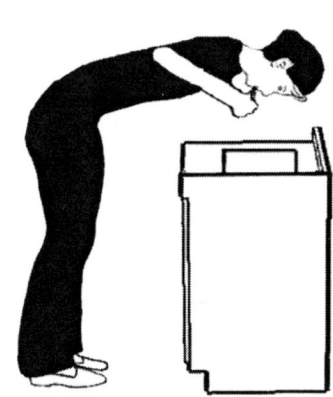

Dressing Tips

General tips for dressing:

- Allow plenty of time for dressing. Hurrying can lead to stress and frustration which can slow you down.
- Sit down when dressing. Choose a chair with firm support and arms.
- Do not sit on the edge of the bed to dress because this can lead to loss of balance and falling.
- Choose clothing with fewer buttons, zippers, and other closures that might be difficult to use.
- Replace buttons by sewing on touch fasteners such as Velcro®. Try loose fitting clothing made of stretchy fabric which is easy to put on.
- Bedroom slippers which can slide off your feet should be replaced with non-skid socks.
- Lightweight, supportive shoes with Velcro® closures, elastic shoelaces, or "curly fries" shoelaces make it easier to put on and take off shoes.
- An extra-long shoehorn helps shoes slide on without your having to bend over.

Remember to think about your body mechanics while dressing. For example; when putting on your shoes avoid rounding forward, and instead either bring a foot up to your knee or put your foot on a footstool.

Correct
Back straight, shoulders down.

Correct
Bringing your leg up instead of bending forward.

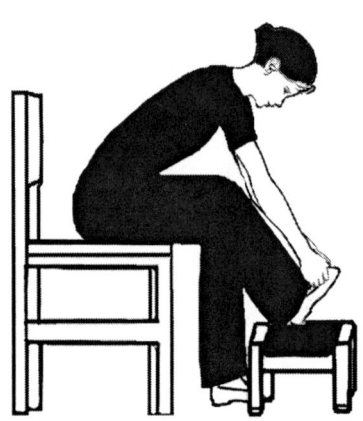
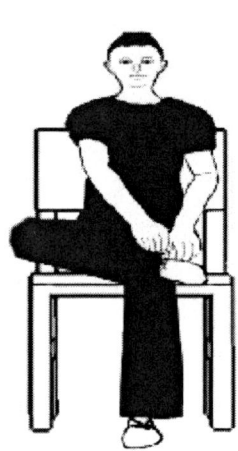

Incorrect
Back and shoulders rounded forward.

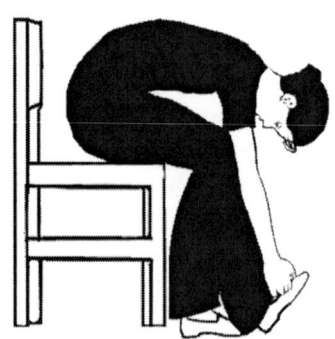

Performing Household Tasks Safely

During housework and yard work it is easy to slip into poor postural habits. Below are some guidelines to help you maintain posture and avoid falls.

- It is safer and easier to push rather than pull.
- If standing for long periods at a sink, counter, or workbench, try putting one foot up on a stool.
- When vacuuming, sweeping, or raking, always face your work. Nose, knees, and toes should all be facing in the same direction. Try to avoid twisting and bending in order to protect your back. Use a rocking motion transferring weight from one foot to the other, thereby relying on your body weight to do the work instead of your back.

Correct
Back straight; knees bent. Broom is close to body, facing work.

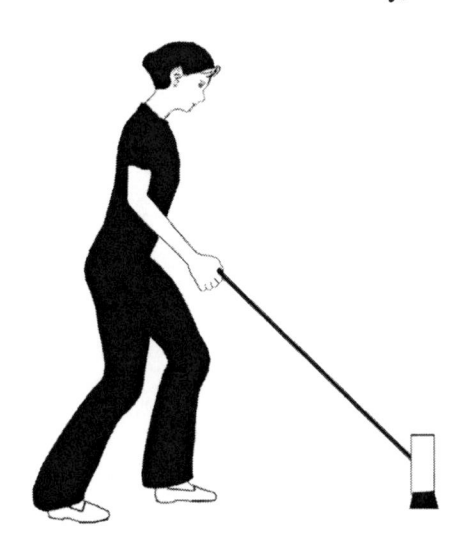

Incorrect
Back and shoulders rounded, knees locked.
Broom too far away.

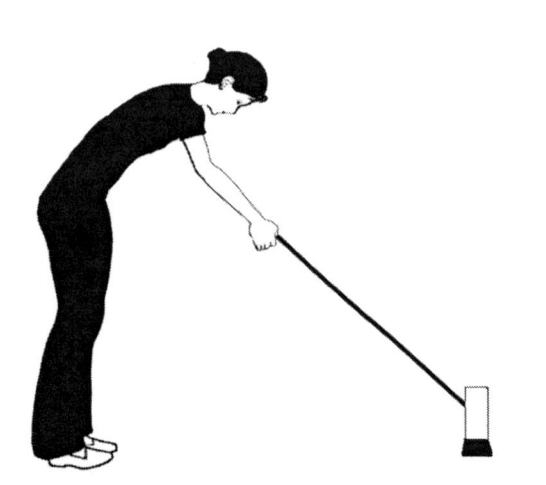

Incorrect
Twisting back and knees.
Nose, knees, and toes not facing work.

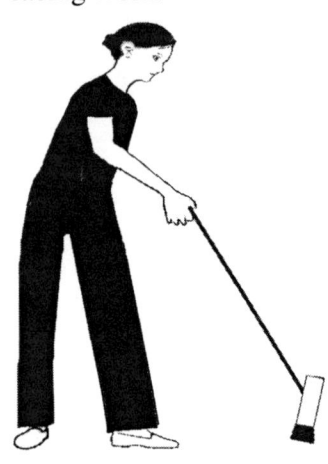

Correct way to sit at computer.

Correct
Back straight, shoulders down.
Screen at eye level.

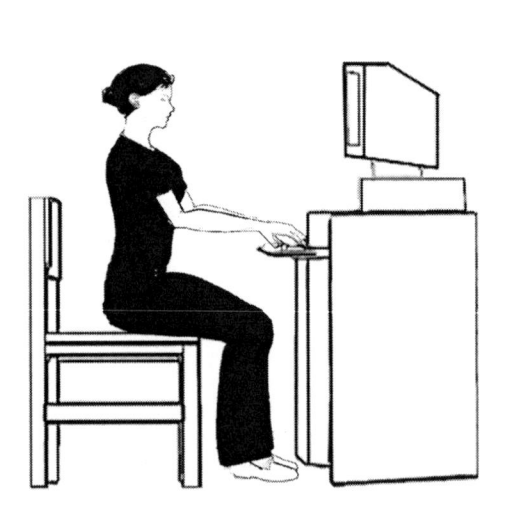

Incorrect
Neck and wrists bent
Screen too high

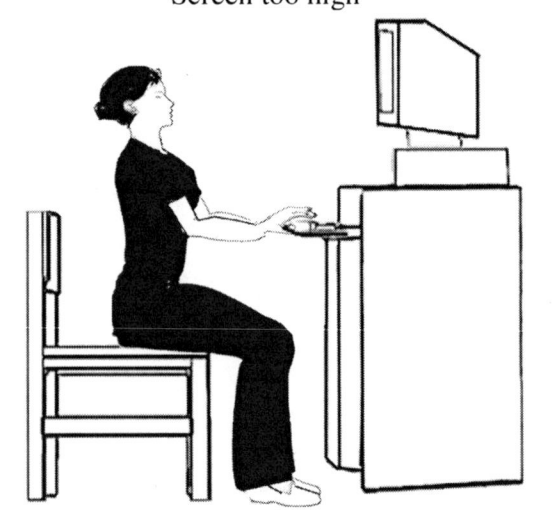

Lifting

When lifting always bend your knees and lift with your legs, not your back. Always test the weight of the object you are going to lift. Keep the object close to your body, and again face your work. Remember to use the hip hinge (pg. 18). Instead of rounding through the back, bend the knees, and reach the buttocks back (as if you were about to sit in a chair). Feet can be about hip width apart or wider if needed for balance. Use this motion regardless of how heavy or light the object is. Many back injuries occur just by moving the wrong way or when lifting light objects!

Correct
Back straight, bending at hips.
Stand close to the object and use your legs to lift.

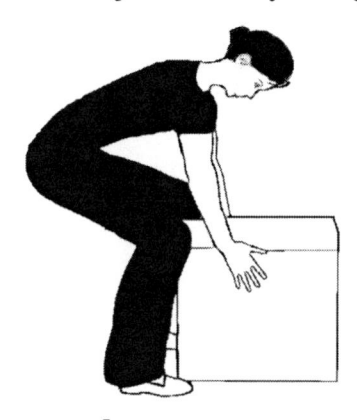

Incorrect
Back rounded, bending at waist. Object too far away, using back to lift.

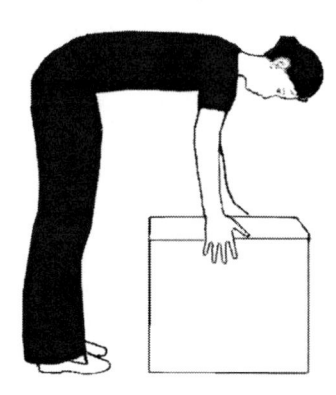

Correct
Correct way to carry. Keep item close to your body.

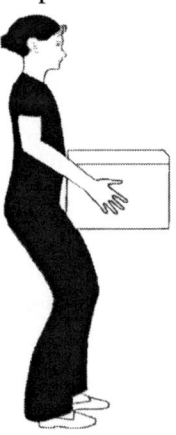

Correct way to reach items in low places.
Get down and close to the object.

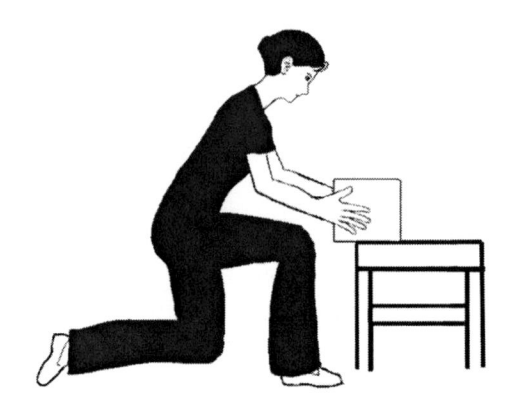

Another way to pick items up off the floor is the golfer's reach. Make sure you hold onto something sturdy to avoid losing your balance. Tip the upper body forward as you lift the back leg. This keeps your back straight versus bending and rounding the back.

It is also important to think about how you reach items that are higher up. If an item is above shoulder height it is best to use a sturdy step stool.

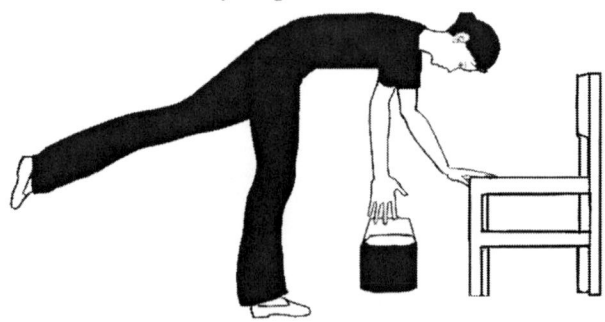

Incorrect

Overreaching from the shoulder, not a sturdy stance. Increased risk for falling backwards or dropping the item.

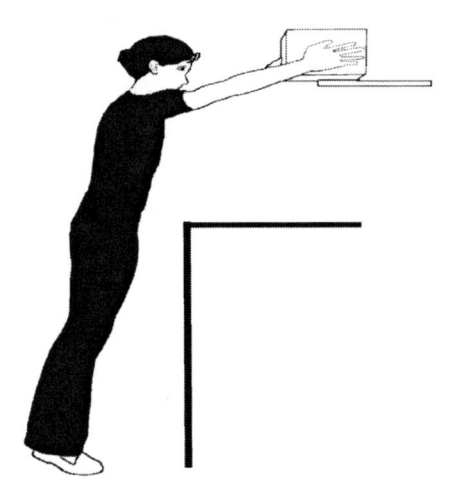

Correct

Place the item on a counter before stepping onto or off of the stool. *Avoid* climbing up or stepping down with items in your hands! Keep the item close to you and get as close as you can to the shelf.

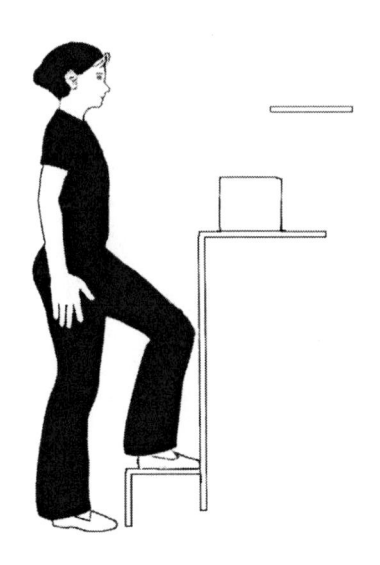

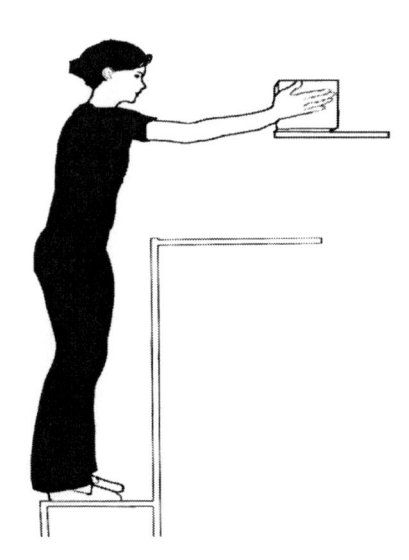

Getting Down on the Floor

If you practice getting up and down from the floor on a regular basis, you will be more likely to be able to get up without help should you fall. People who fall at home must sometimes wait hours or even days before help arrives. When first attempting this, make sure you have someone around to help you until you can easily get up alone. Below are the steps to take to safely get down onto the floor.

1. First make sure there is a sturdy chair nearby. Use the hip hinge motion (pg. 18) to place your hands on the chair.

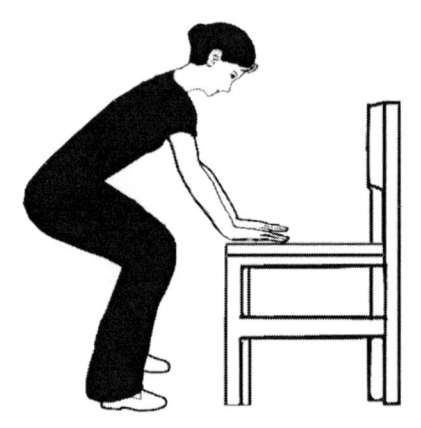

2. Then place one knee (whichever knee is more comfortable to do this with) on the floor. Continue to use the chair for support.

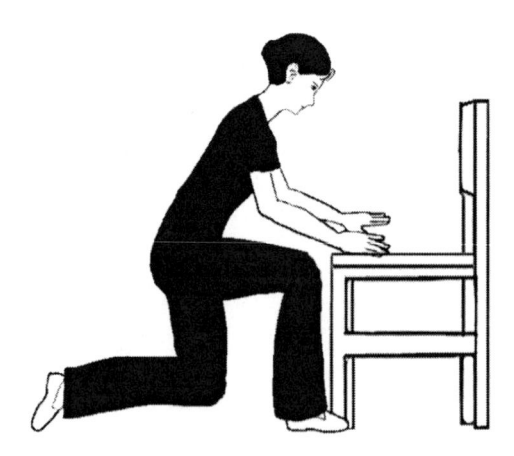

3. Then come down on to all fours and move the chair away a bit.

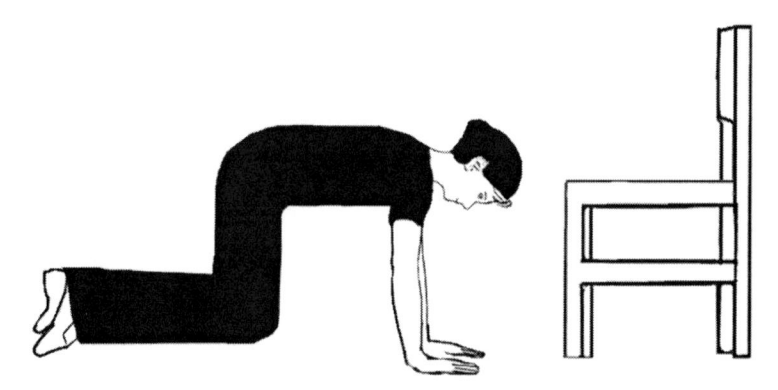

4. Then lower yourself down onto one hip, whichever hip is more comfortable to bear weight on.

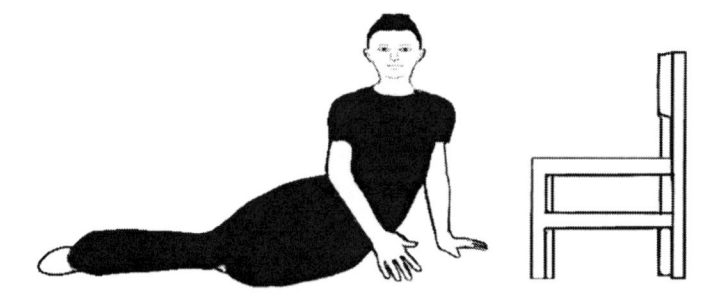

5. Next, lower yourself down so that you are lying on your side.

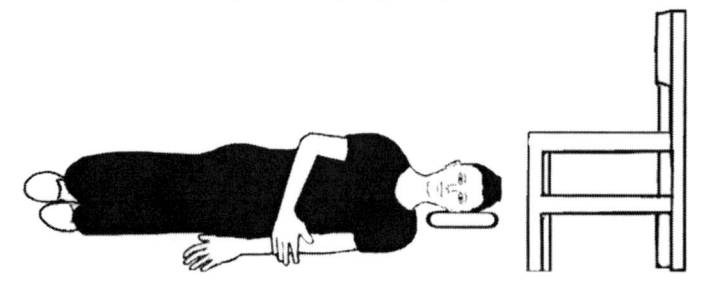

6. From here you can roll over onto your back.

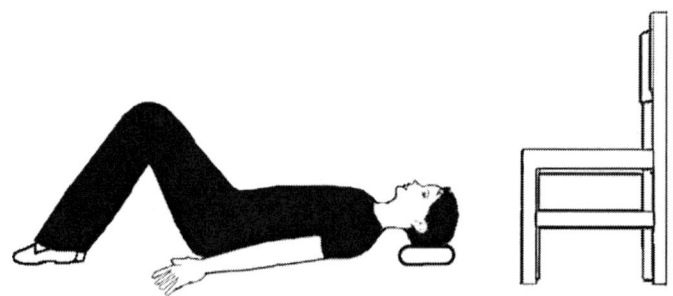

Getting Up From the Floor

Below are the steps to take to safely get up from the floor.

1. Make sure there is a chair or sturdy piece of furniture near by. If you have fallen in the middle of the room, crawl or scoot yourself over to something sturdy.

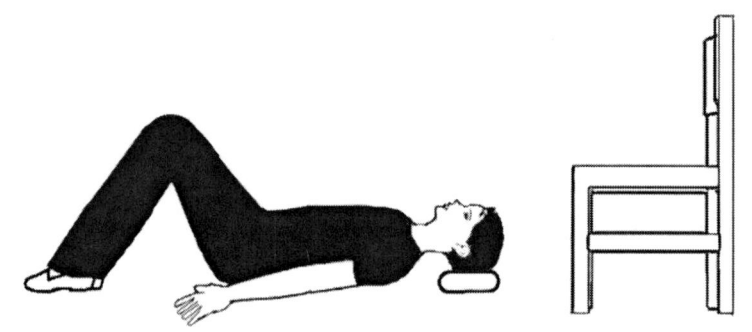

2. If you are on your back, first roll onto one side, (whichever side is more comfortable to bear weight on).

3. Roll your body as a unit, the same as when getting out of bed.

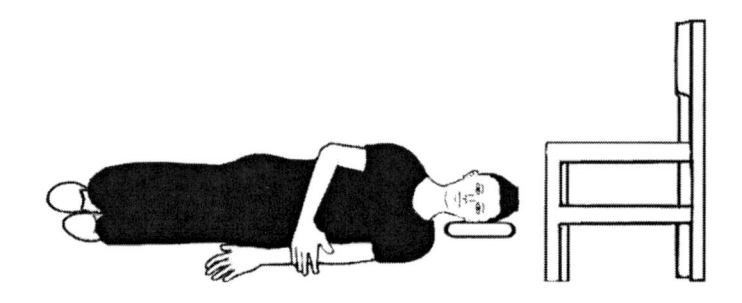

4. Then, using your arms, push up onto your hip.

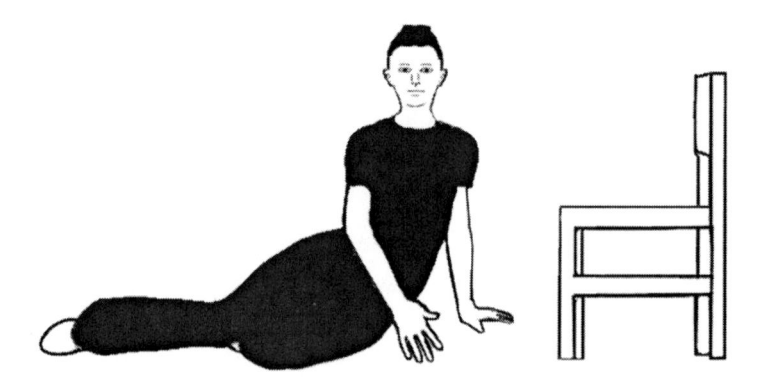

5. Next come up to all fours.

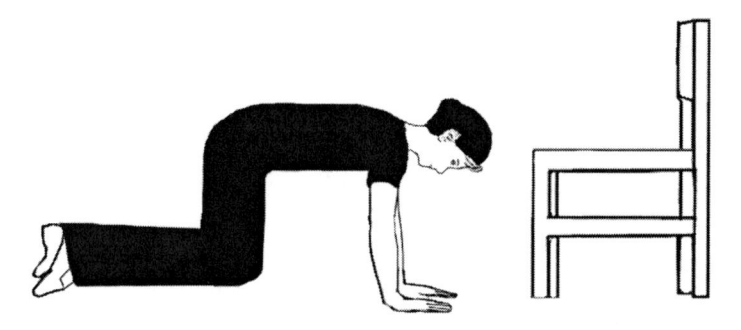

6. Bring one foot forward so that you are on one knee (whichever knee is more comfortable to do this with). Place your hands on the chair for support. If you are outside or not near a chair push off of your thigh.

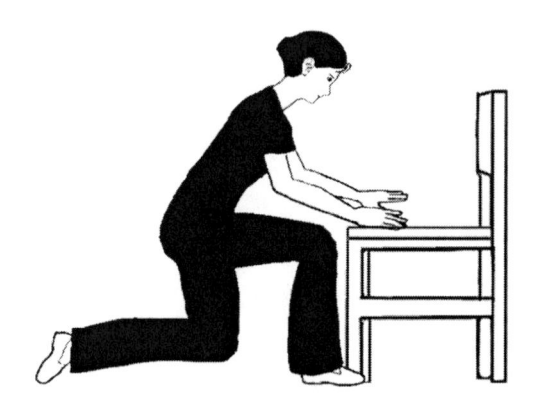

7. Using your arms on the chair or your thigh, hip hinge up to standing. Use the hip hinge motion and avoid rounding your back.

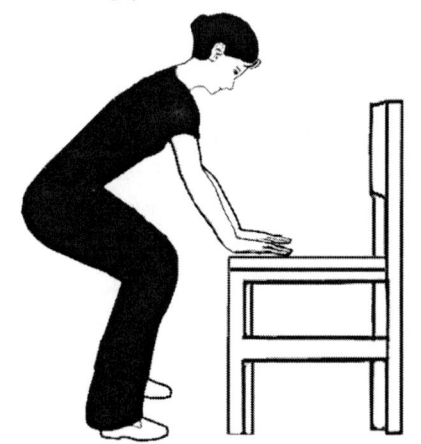

Begin to incorporate correct body mechanics techniques on a daily basis. At first it may seem like daily tasks take longer, but with more practice using correct body mechanics will become more natural. With time, you may find that you automatically correct yourself, and eventually it will become common practice to use good working habits.

To fully manage your symptoms and remain active, using correct body mechanics is an important step. Taking the time to do things correctly and safely will help to reduce the risk of falls and keep your back and joints safe from injury. Many falls and accidents happen as the result of rushing and not thinking our actions through. Taking the time to do things correctly helps avoid accidents enabling you to stay independent longer.

If you are experiencing significant difficulty with any of your daily activities, talk with your health care provider about attending physical or occupational therapy. Physical and occupational therapists are specially trained to work with you and your individual situation to help make everyday activities safer and more enjoyable.

> "I used to always worry about falling. I not only worried about getting hurt but also about how I was going to get back up. I sometimes would fall when alone at home or outside in the driveway. It was embarrassing as I would have to wait for someone to help me get back up. After participating in the exercises in this book, and by following the instructions on getting up from the floor, I no longer have to wait for assistance to get up. I now have the strength, balance and know how to help myself." - J.M. Massachusetts

Chapter Two
Diaphragmatic Breathing and Warm Up Exercises

"A journey of a thousand miles begins with a single step."
-Confucius

   Before beginning any exercise routine it is important to "warm-up" the body. "Warming-up" simply means preparing the joints and muscles for movement, and allowing the heart and breathing rate to increase slowly. If you do not take the time to warm up the body correctly you risk injury to the joints and muscles.

   With Parkinson's disease there is often an increase in rigidity and stiffness of the body. Therefore, it is helpful to do some gentle range of motion exercises to prepare the body for more strenuous exercise. The following exercises help loosen the joints and muscles and increase the delivery of oxygen, which makes the body more receptive to aerobic, strength training, and flexibility exercises.

Diaphragmatic Breathing

   Before beginning to explore different movement techniques it is important to discuss breathing. Most people take shallow breaths moving only the chest and shoulders. When taking shallow breaths the diaphragm is not used to it's full capacity. It is more efficient and beneficial to learn to breathe more deeply, using the diaphragm and the abdominal cavity. This is especially important as Parkinson's disease can cause a decrease in lung capacity which can lead to speech becoming soft and difficult for others to hear. Learning to breathe more deeply increases lung capacity and improves voice projection. Learning to breathe abdominally (from the diaphragm) also helps to promote relaxation, which improves physical and mental health. This occurs since belly breathing is a more efficient way for the body to take in oxygen and remove carbon dioxide with the least effort.

   The diaphragm is a large, dome-shaped muscle that contracts rhythmically and continually, and most of the time involuntarily. The diaphragm sits beneath the lungs and above the abdominal cavity. When you exhale the abdominal muscles should contract, allowing the diaphragm to move upward, so the air is fully expelled from the lungs.

When breathing in the abdominal muscles relax and move outwards, allowing the diaphragm muscle to move downward so that the lungs can expand.

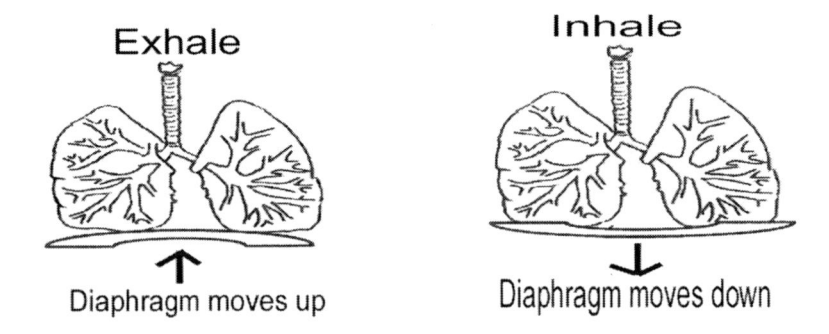

Though breathing is an automatic function, the movements of the diaphragm can be controlled voluntarily with training. Benefits of diaphragmatic breathing include:

- A more efficient exchange of oxygen and carbon dioxide
- Improved circulation
- Removal of waste products from the blood
- Slower heart rate and breathing rate
- Calming of the mind

This method of breathing may feel awkward because we were often taught to pull in the stomach muscles as we inhale, but this actually restricts the movement of the diaphragm. However, with practice this deeper form of breathing will become more natural. The easiest way to practice diaphragmatic breathing is lying down, the second easiest is while standing, and the most difficult is while seated. You can begin to try this deep breathing by lying on your bed or couch. Then try it while standing, and then seated. We will use this breath during every exercise and movement in this book. This breathing technique should be done as much as possible through the nose rather than the mouth. Breathing through the nose is more efficient and relaxing for the body, because the nasal cavity is better designed to purify and warm the air. If you are experiencing any type of respiratory or sinus concerns, or if you become dizzy while breathing strictly through the nose, try inhaling only through the nose and then exhaling through pursed lips.

How to do Belly Breathing Lying Down

Lie on your back with a pillow under your head if needed. Place one hand on your belly. As you exhale through the nose gently contract the abdominal muscles and push all of the air out of your belly and lungs. The hand on the belly should move down. Think of moving the belly towards the floor.

Exhale: Belly pulls in pushing the air out

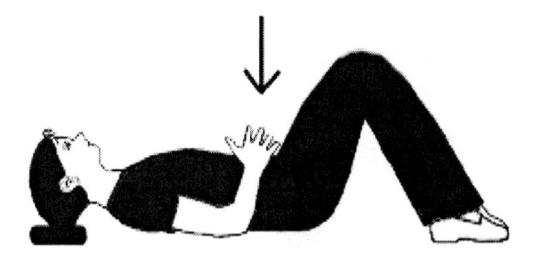

As you inhale through the nose let the abdominal muscles relax and let the belly rise first. With the inhalation the hand on the belly should move up. Think of moving the belly towards the ceiling. Then let the chest rise. It may take some practice to have the belly move first, or at all.

Inhale: Belly expands taking air in

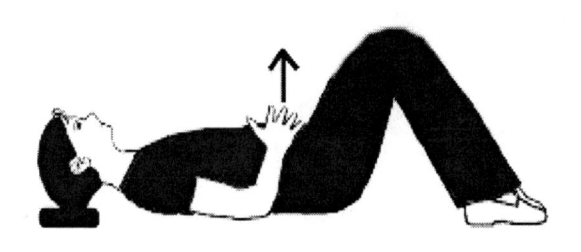

How to do Belly Breathing Seated

Sit away from the back of the chair with your feet flat on the floor. The shoulders stay down and relaxed. Place one hand on your belly. As you exhale through the nose, gently contract your abdominal muscles and push all of the air out of your belly and lungs. The hand on your belly should move inwards. Think of moving your belly towards the back of the chair.

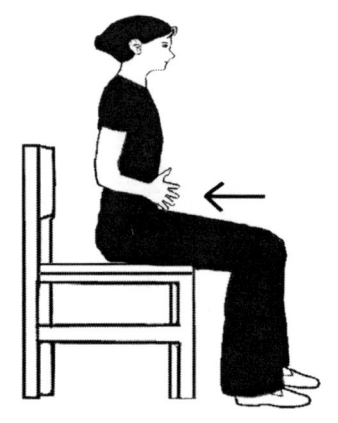

As you inhale through the nose let the belly rise first. Your belly and the hand on your belly should move outwards with the inhalation. Then let the chest rise. It may take some practice to have the belly move first, or at all. Keep the shoulders down and relaxed the entire time.

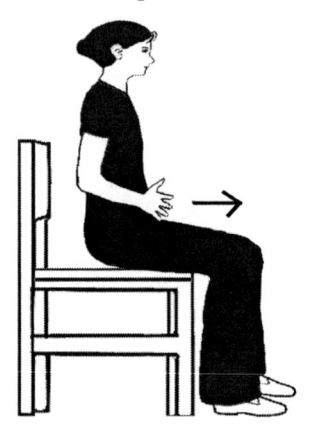

"I used to find myself getting out of breath during everyday activities and I was having trouble speaking loudly enough for my husband to hear me. I stared practicing the deep diaphragmatic breathing exercises for fifteen minutes everyday. At my last appointment my doctor told me that my lung capacity has improved by fifteen percent. Practicing deep breathing exercises helped me gain some control over my PD."   - M.D. Massachusetts.

Warm Up/Range of Motion Exercises

The following movements should be done slowly and gently, allowing the body to prepare for more vigorous movements. Perform each movement eight to twelve times. Without forcing, try to increase your range of motion with each repetition. Do not push your body to do more than feels right.

Since each day with Parkinson's can be different, each exercise session will be as well. Use the warm-up segment as an opportunity to notice which areas of your body are tight or uncomfortable, and which areas move more easily. This process will help you to determine which components of the exercise regimen would be appropriate to do, and how vigorous or gently you should proceed.

Warm-up exercises should always be done before any of the other segments. We encourage you to do all of the warm-ups listed as each one targets a specific area of the body and a specific type of joint movement.

Half Neck Rolls

This exercise loosens the muscles of the neck. Sit up straight at the front edge of the chair. If you are experiencing discomfort or find yourself slouching, slide all the way back in the chair so your back remains straight.

| Drop your right ear to your right shoulder. | Circle your chin to your chest. | Circle your left ear to your left shoulder. |

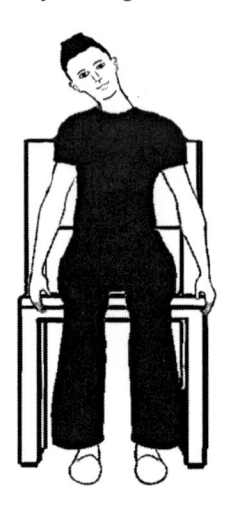

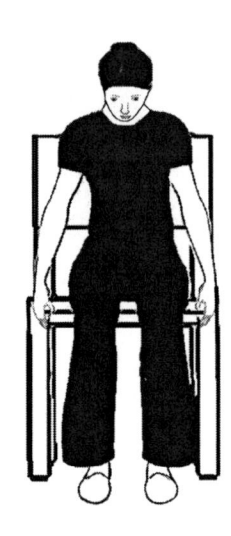

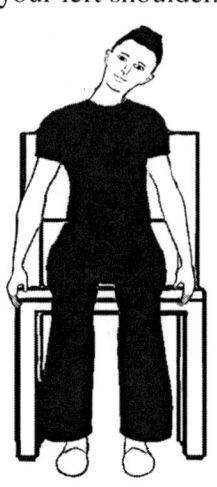

Reverse the movement making a half circle from left to right. It is not recommended to drop the head backwards as this compresses the neck. Exhale as you circle your chin to your chest and inhale as you roll the ear to the shoulder. Use deep belly breathing through just the nose as much as possible. Do this movement *slowly and gently,* counting *one-one thousand, two-one thousand, three-one thousand, four-one thousand* each time you circle your chin to your chest, and use the same count each time you roll the ear to the shoulder. Do this movement eight to twelve times. One repetition involves going to both sides.

Checklist
- ✓ Sit up straight
- ✓ Do not turn the head or drop the head to the back
- ✓ Move slowly using a "four thousand count" for each movement
- ✓ Exhale as you circle the chin to the chest, and inhale as you roll the ear to the shoulder
- ✓ Use diaphragmatic breathing through the nose as much as possible
- ✓ Do not exercise to the point of strain or discomfort

Neck Stretch

Hold to the right, dropping the right ear to the right shoulder. Do not turn your head or chin, look straight forward to stretch the side of the neck. Each time you exhale let the right ear drop closer to the right shoulder and gently press the left shoulder down a bit more. Hold for five to ten deep belly breaths.

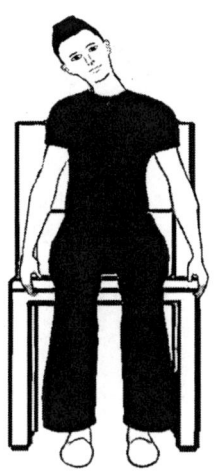

Next, hold to the left side, dropping the left ear to the left shoulder. Do not turn your head or chin, look straight forward to stretch the side of the neck. Each time you exhale let the left ear drop closer to the left shoulder and gently press the right shoulder down a bit more. Hold for five to ten deep belly breaths.

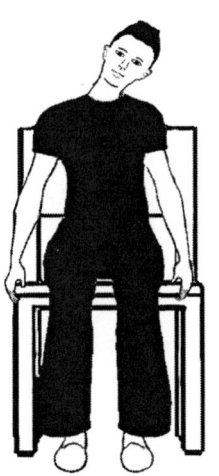

Next, drop the chin to the chest, and hold. Sit up straight. With each exhale roll the shoulders back and down and gently drop the chin, stretching the back of the neck. Hold for five to ten deep belly breaths.

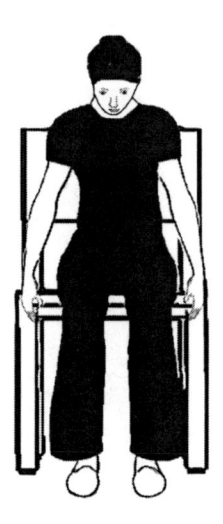

Checklist
- ✓ Sit up straight
- ✓ Do not turn the head, look straight forward
- ✓ Move slowly using a "four thousand count" for each movement
- ✓ Hold each stretch for five to ten deep belly breaths
- ✓ Use diaphragmatic breathing through the nose as much as possible
- ✓ Do not exercise to the point of strain or discomfort

Head Rotation

Bring the head back to a neutral position. Check to see that you are still sitting up straight and away from the back of the chair if possible.

Keeping your chin parallel to the floor, turn your head to the right to look over the right shoulder. Come back to center. Then turn the head to the left and look over the left shoulder. Come back to center. Exhale each time you turn the head to the side. Inhale each time you come back to center. Do this movement *slowly and gently,* counting *one-one thousand, two-one thousand, three-one thousand, four-one thousand* each time you turn to the side. Use the same count as you come back to the center. Do this movement eight to twelve times. One repetition involves going to both sides.

Turning the head to the right.   Turning the head to the left.

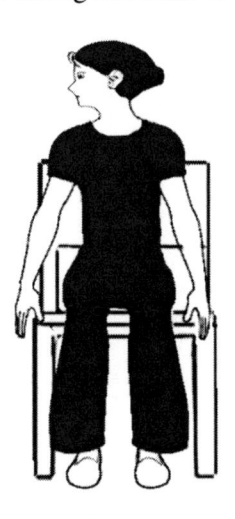

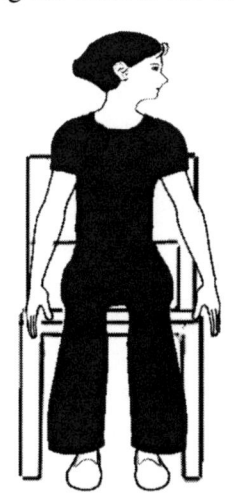

Checklist
- ✓ Sit up straight
- ✓ Move slowly using a "four thousand count" for each movement
- ✓ Use diaphragmatic breathing through the nose as much as possible
- ✓ Do not exercise to the point of strain or discomfort

Head Rotation Stretch

After completing eight to twelve repetitions. Hold to the right side looking over the right shoulder. Each time you exhale see if you can look a bit more to the right and gently press the left shoulder back a bit more. Hold for five to ten deep belly breaths.

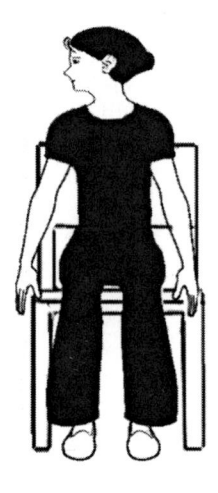

Repeat on the left side.

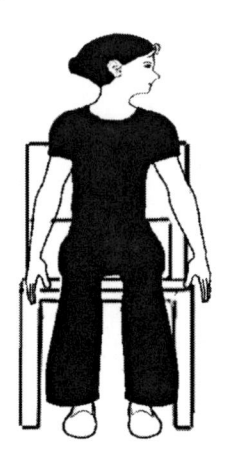

Checklist
- ✓ Sit up straight
- ✓ Hold each stretch for five to ten deep belly breaths
- ✓ Use diaphragmatic breathing through the nose as much as possible
- ✓ Do not exercise to the point of strain or discomfort

Chin Tuck

This movement should be done gently just a few times. This exercise helps to strengthen the muscles in the back of the neck. This will help to correct the forward head position common in those with Parkinson's disease.

Bring the head to a neutral position. Check to see if you are still sitting up straight and away from the back of the chair if possible. Keeping the chin parallel to the floor, gently retract or draw the chin back straightening the back of the neck. Exhale as you draw the head back and inhale as you release forward. Do this movement *slowly and gently*, counting *one-one thousand, two-one thousand, three-one thousand, four-one thousand* each time you draw the chin back. Use the same count as you release the chin forward. Repeat eight to twelve times.

Neutral position   Draw the chin straight back

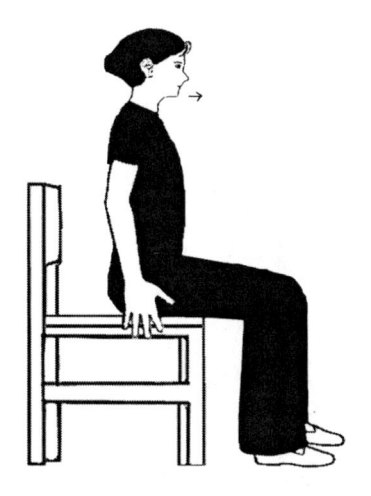

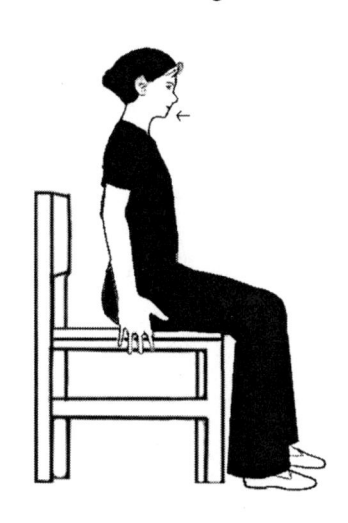

Checklist
- ✓ Sit up straight
- ✓ Move slowly using a "four thousand count" for each movement
- ✓ Keep the chin parallel to the floor
- ✓ Use diaphragmatic breathing through the nose as much as possible
- ✓ Do not exercise to the point of strain or discomfort

Shoulder Rolls

Bring the head back to a neutral position. Check to see if you are still sitting up straight and away from the back of the chair if possible.

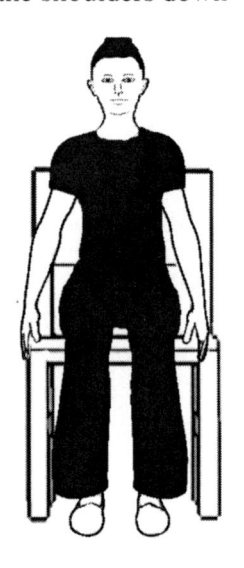

Lift the shoulders up towards the ears as high as you can in a shrugging motion. Then roll the shoulders down and back, pressing them down as far as you can. Do this movement *slowly and gently,* counting *one-one thousand, two-one thousand, three-one thousand, four-one thousand* each time you lift the shoulders. Use the same count as you lower the shoulders. Repeat for eight to twelve shoulder rolls. Inhale as you lift the shoulders up and exhale as you press the shoulders down. Exaggerate at both ends of the movement. Make sure you do not bend the elbows. The arms stay straight and the movement is all in the shoulders. This is an area which becomes stiff for those with Parkinson's, so it is helpful to have someone watch you do this movement to make sure the shoulders are both lifting up and pressing down.

Press the shoulders down	Lift the shoulders up

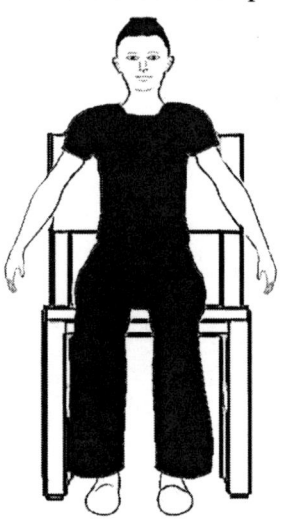

Checklist
- ✓ Sit up straight
- ✓ Use diaphragmatic breathing through the nose as much as possible
- ✓ Move slowly using a "four thousand count" for each movement
- ✓ Make sure you are lifting the shoulders up and lowering them down
- ✓ Do not bend the elbows, keep the arms straight
- ✓ Do not exercise to the point of strain or discomfort

Seated Spinal Twist

This movement will help to loosen the trunk muscles. If you have any sensitivities or injuries in your back such as osteoporosis or fractures you may wish to check with your health care provider about the appropriateness of twisting movements. Feeling a stretch or pull in the muscles can mean that you are stretching them, but you should never experience sharp or stabbing pain either during or after your exercise session. It is recommended that you do this movement very slowly with control and be aware of how it affects you. Remember, *never* go to the point of pain.

Sit up straight and away from the back of the chair if possible. Hold onto your elbows, keep the shoulders down away from the ears, and sit up straight. Begin to turn to the right, *turning at your waist.* Bring your arms and head with you. Turn to look over your right shoulder as far as you can. Come back to center and repeat to the left.

Do this movement *slowly and gently,* counting *one-one thousand, two-one thousand, three-one thousand, four-one thousand* each time you turn to the side. Use the same count as you turn back to the center. Inhale as you come to the center, and exhale as you turn to the side. Do this movement eight to twelve times. One repetition involves going to both sides.

Gently turn to the right, looking over your right shoulder.

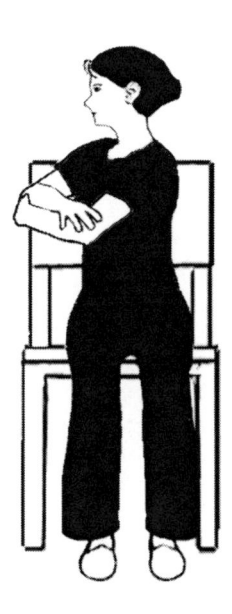

Come back to center.   Gently turn to the left, looking over
                                              your left shoulder

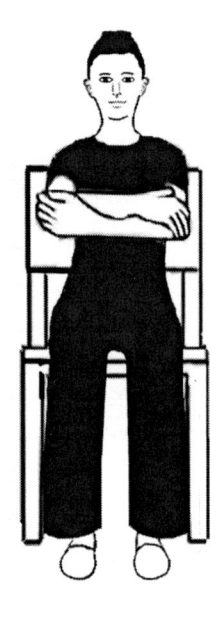

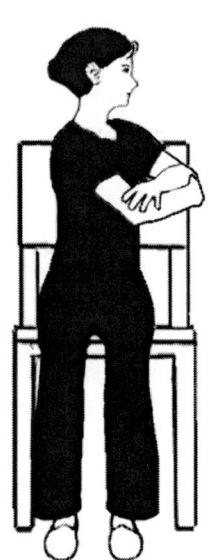

Checklist
- ✓ Sit up straight
- ✓ Use caution with twisting movements if you have back injuries or sensitivities
- ✓ Move slowly using a "four thousand count" for each movement
- ✓ Make sure you turn from the waist, not just the shoulders
- ✓ Turn your head to look back over your shoulder to complete the movement
- ✓ Use diaphragmatic breathing through the nose as much as possible
- ✓ Keep the shoulders down and back
- ✓ Do not exercise to the point of strain or discomfort

Seated Spinal Stretch

Comeback to center. Press the shoulders down away from the ears and sit up straight. Begin to turn by *turning at your waist*. Bring your arms and head with you. Turn to look over your right shoulder as far as you can and hold. Each time you inhale sit up straighter. Each time you exhale see if you can turn and see a bit further behind you. Keep checking that the shoulders have not lifted up towards the ears. Hold for five to ten deep belly breaths. Repeat holding the stretch to the left.

Hold to the right   Hold to the left

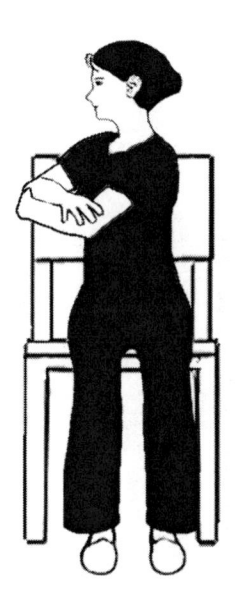

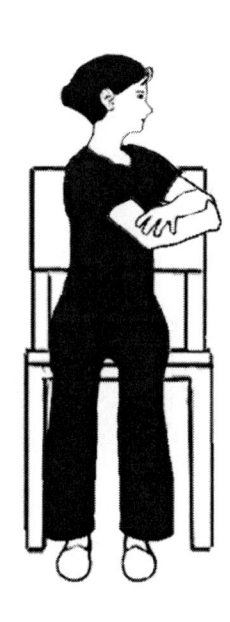

Checklist
- ✓ Sit up straight
- ✓ Use caution with twisting movements if you have back injuries or sensitivities
- ✓ Hold to each side for five to ten deep belly breaths
- ✓ Make sure you turn from the waist, not just the shoulders
- ✓ Turn your head to look back over your shoulder to complete the movement
- ✓ Use diaphragmatic breathing through the nose as much as possible
- ✓ Keep the shoulders down and back
- ✓ Do not exercise to the point of strain or discomfort

Seated Cat Stretch

This stretch loosens the low back muscles. The low back is an area that often becomes tight and prone to injury. Since it can be a difficult area to learn to isolate, it is helpful to have someone watch to see if you are performing the movement correctly. A common mistake is to just lean back with the whole body instead of rounding the low back. Check that you are sitting up straight and away from the back of the chair. For this exercise, you need to be at the very front edge of the seat in order to have room to move the low back. First push the abdomen forward and the shoulders back to create an arch in the low back. Do not drop the head back. Next, let the shoulders round forward, pull the abdominal muscles in, and let the low back round out. Think of a cat arching its back. Again, it is your low back, not the upper back or shoulders, that is moving closer to the back of the chair.

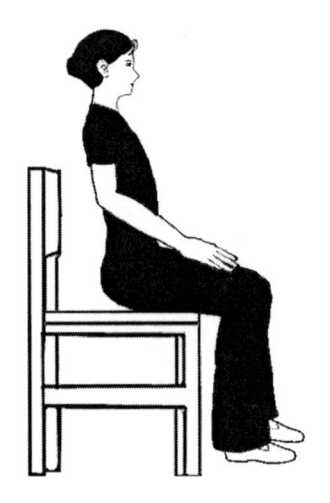

Arch the back   Round the low back

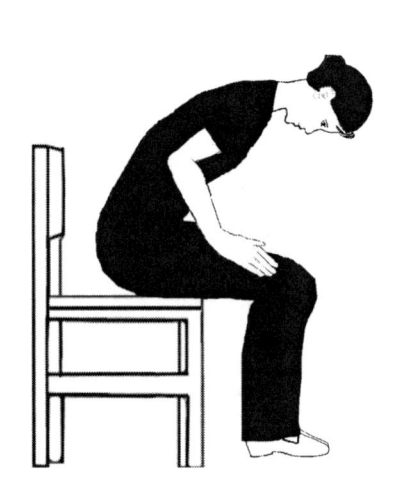

Go back and forth between arching and rounding the low back. Inhale as you arch, and exhale as you round. Do this movement *slowly and gently,* counting *one-one thousand, two-one thousand, three-one thousand, four-one thousand* as you round back, and use the same count each time you arch the back. Do this movement eight to twelve times.

Checklist
- ✓ Move slowly using a "four thousand count" for each movement
- ✓ Use diaphragmatic breathing through the nose as much as possible
- ✓ Make sure you are isolating and rounding the low back and not just leaning back with the whole body
- ✓ Do not exercise to the point of strain or discomfort

Chest Opener

This movement stretches the shoulders and opens the chest. If you have any sensitivities in your shoulders do this movement gently. Check that you are sitting up straight and away from the back of the chair if possible. Clasp your hands behind your head. Do not pull the head forward. Use the chin tuck exercise to keep your neck in alignment. If you can not bring your hands behind your neck, you can bring your fingertips to the sides of your head. As you continue these stretches, you may find that your flexibility increases. Bring the elbows together as close you can without pulling the head forward; remember to use good alignment.

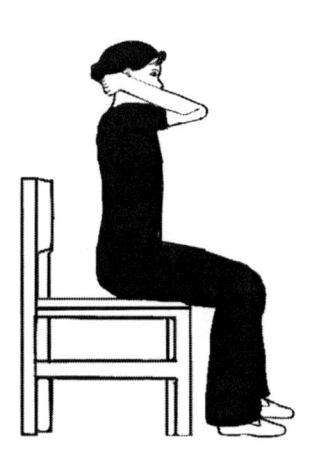

Next, bring the elbows back and open as far as you comfortably can. Let the chest come forward and the low back arch slightly. Gently squeeze the shoulder blades together in the back, and keep the shoulders down away from the ears. Inhale as you open the elbows, and exhale as the elbows come together.

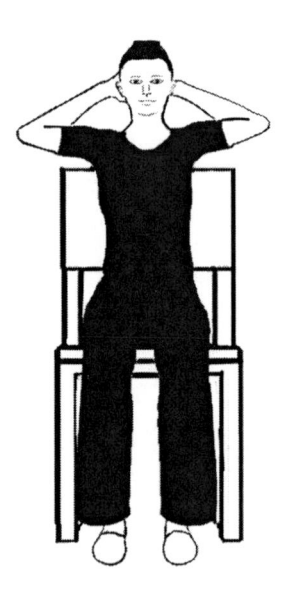

Do this movement *slowly and gently, counting one-one thousand, two-one thousand, three-one thousand, four-one thousand* each time you open the elbows, and use the same count each time you bring the elbows together. Do this movement eight to twelve times. Try to take deep breaths as you bring the elbows back. This movement opens the chest allowing the lungs to fully expand.

> Checklist
> ✓ Sit up straight
> ✓ Move slowly using a "four thousand count" for each movement
> ✓ Use diaphragmatic breathing through the nose as much as possible
> ✓ Do not pull your head forward with your hands
> ✓ Do not exercise to the point of strain or discomfort

Before proceeding to standing movements, it is good to warm up the feet and ankles. These movements are helpful if you have been sitting for some time. Many falls happen while transitioning from sitting to standing. Sitting for long periods can reduce the circulation in the legs, impairing balance. These next two movements will help to restore circulation to the legs.

Toe Lifts

Check that you are sitting up straight and away from the back of the chair if possible. Keeping the heels on the floor, lift both toes off the floor as high as you can. Repeat eight to twelve times.

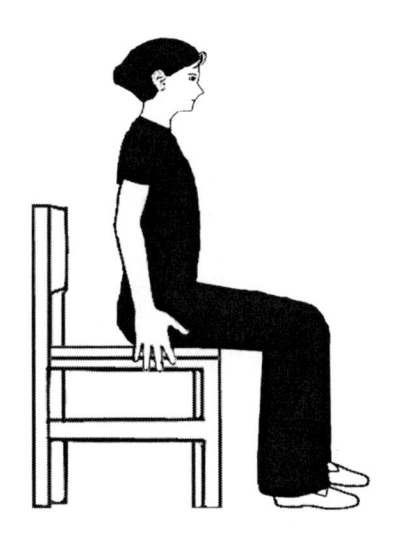

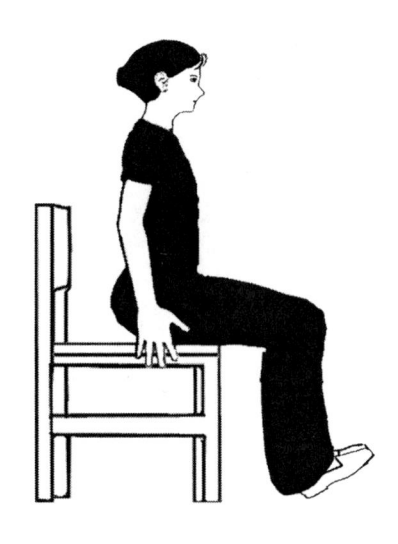

Checklist
✓ Sit up straight
✓ Move slowly using a "four thousand count" for each movement
✓ Use diaphragmatic breathing through the nose as much as possible
✓ Do not exercise to the point of strain or discomfort

Heel Lifts

Check that you are sitting up straight and away from the back of the chair if possible. Keeping the toes on the floor, lift both heels off the floor as high as you can. Repeat eight to twelve times. You can also alternate between these two movements i.e., lift the toes and then the heels, and continue back and forth.

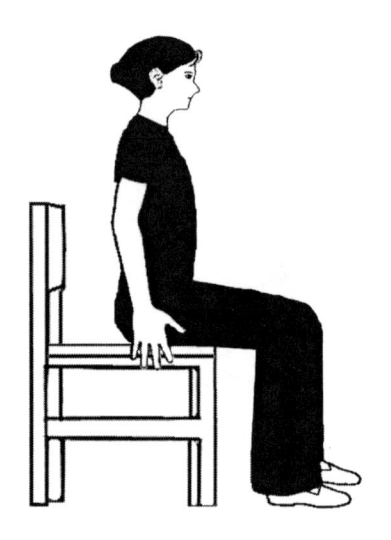

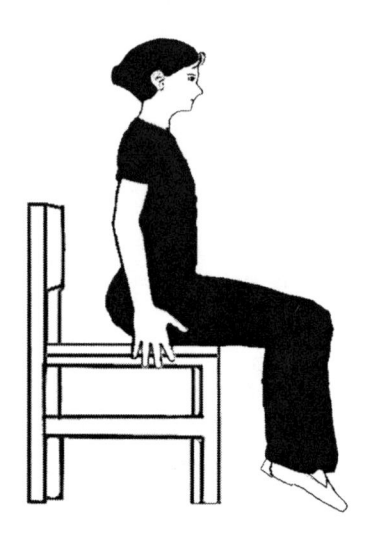

Checklist
- ✓ Sit up straight
- ✓ Move slowly using a "four thousand count" for each movement
- ✓ Use diaphragmatic breathing through the nose as much as possible
- ✓ Do not exercise to the point of strain or discomfort

The next few exercises are illustrated in a standing position, or standing and holding on, to help you to get your balance before moving on to more vigorous exercises. *Do as much as you can standing*, but seated versions are also shown if needed. If you choose to sit, keep checking that you are sitting up straight and away from the back of the chair if possible.

Side Bending

This movement helps to loosen the muscles of the waist. Check your posture before you begin. Shoulders should be back and down and over the hips. Knees should remain slightly bent. Tuck the chin in and think about pushing the crown of the head up to the ceiling without lifting your chin. The abdominal muscles are lightly pulled in, but not so much as to restrict your breathing.

Arms are resting by your sides. Let your right ear drop towards your right shoulder. Then begin to slide your right hand down the outside of the right leg, towards the knee. Be careful that you *do not lean forward* while bending; the shoulders should stay over the hips. Pretend you are between two panes of glass and can only bend sideways, and can not move forward or back.

Inhale as you stand up, and exhale as you bend. Do this movement *slowly and gently*, counting *one-one thousand, two-one thousand, three-one thousand, four-one thousand* each time you bend to the side, and use the same count each time you stand up straight. Do this movement eight to twelve times. One repetition involves going both ways.

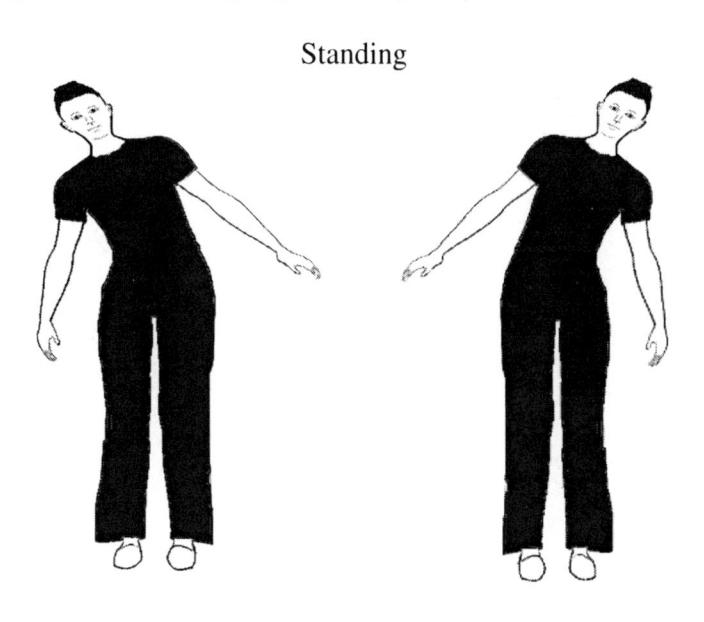

Standing

Standing with assistance

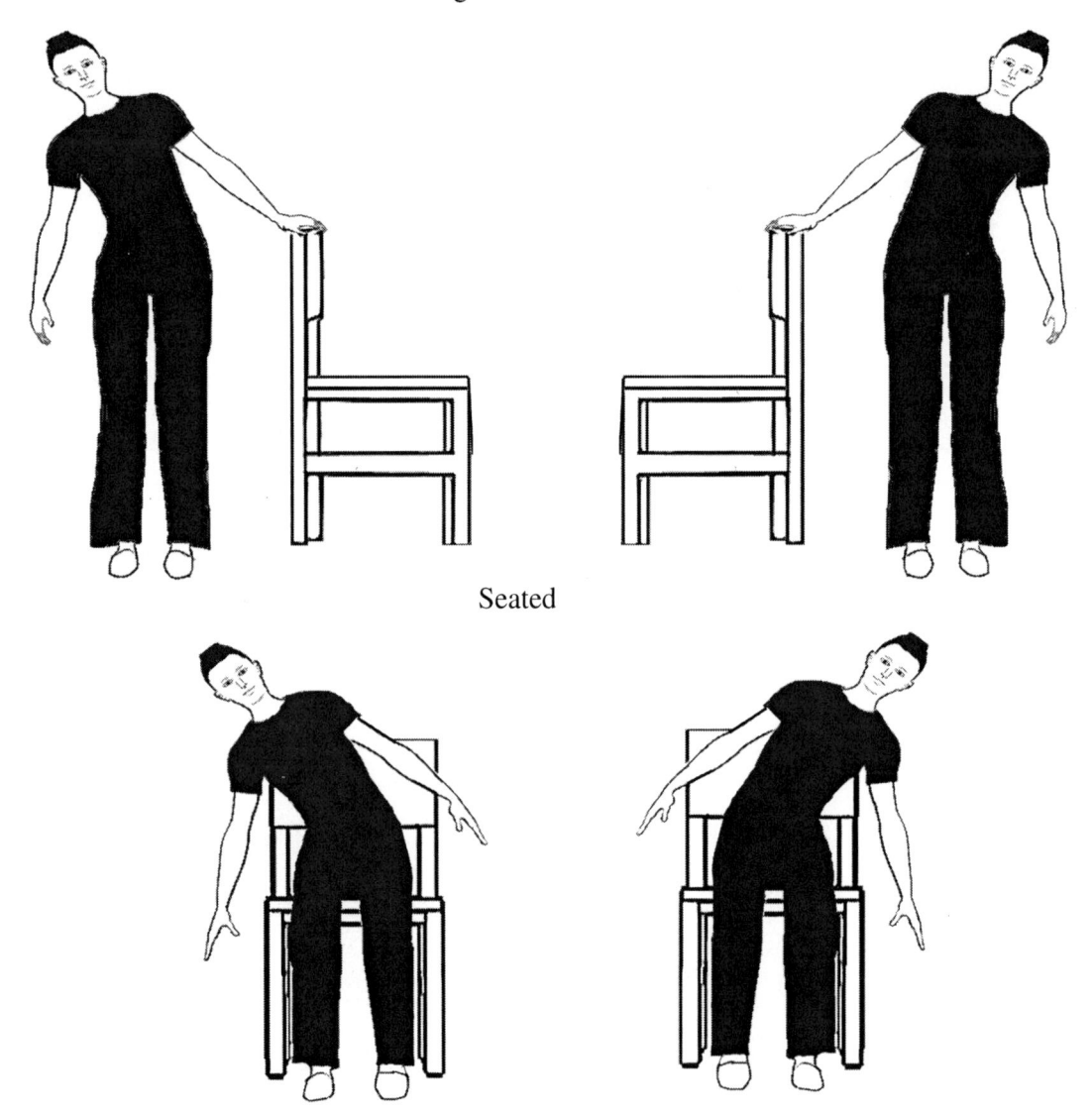

Seated

Checklist
- ✓ Stand or sit up straight
- ✓ Move slowly using a "four thousand count" for each movement
- ✓ Do not lean forward when bending
- ✓ Keep the shoulders over the hips
- ✓ Use diaphragmatic breathing through the nose as much as possible
- ✓ When standing keep the knees slightly bent
- ✓ Do not exercise to the point of strain or discomfort

Side Stretch

Next, slide down and hold the stretch to the right side. Bring your left arm up overhead. *Do not lean forward,* keep the shoulders over the hips. Do not let the top arm come forward, keep it over your head. Bring the left elbow as close to the left ear as you can. Each time you exhale see if you can slide your right hand further down your leg, and bring your left elbow closer to your ear. Hold for five to ten deep belly breaths.

Come back to center, check your posture, then hold to the left side. Each time you exhale see if you can slide your left hand further down your leg, and bring your right elbow closer to your ear. Hold for five to ten deep belly breaths.

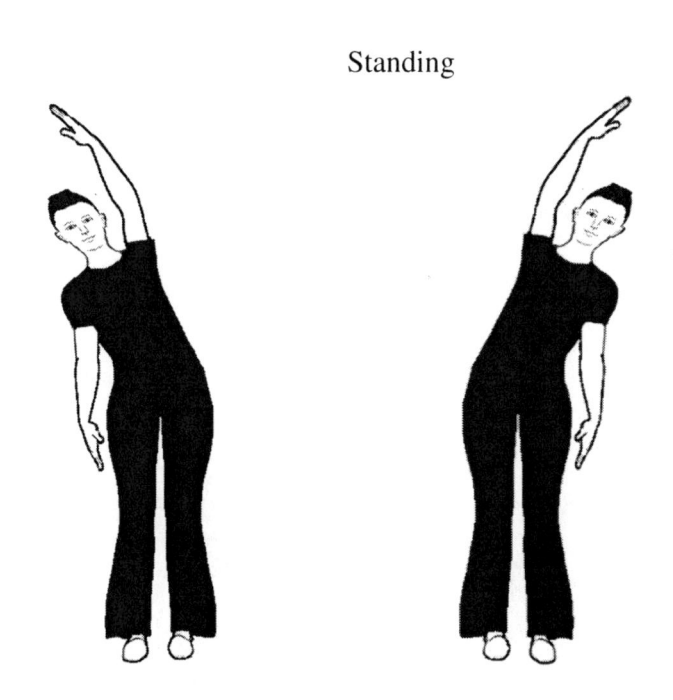

Standing

Standing with assistance

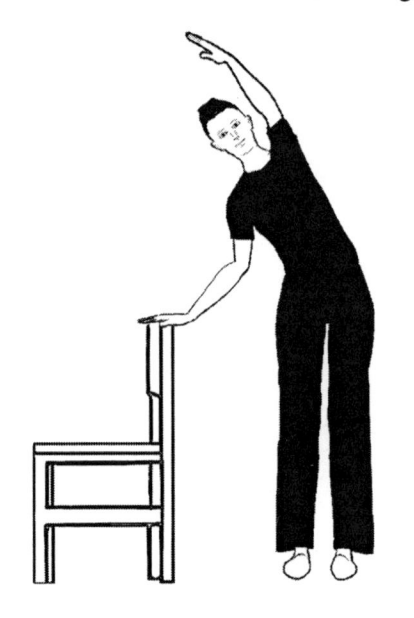

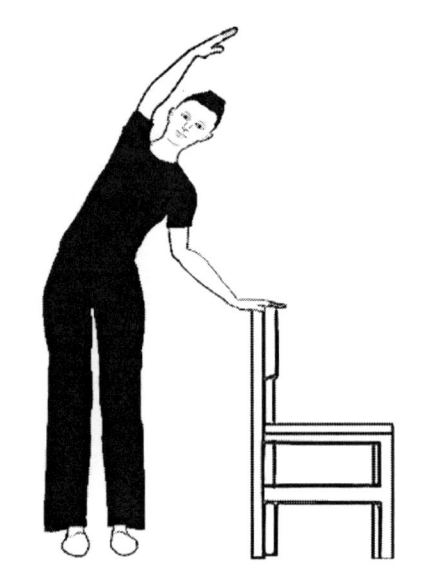

Seated

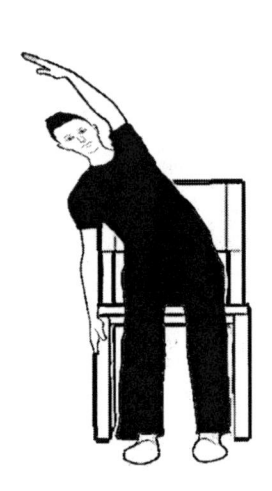

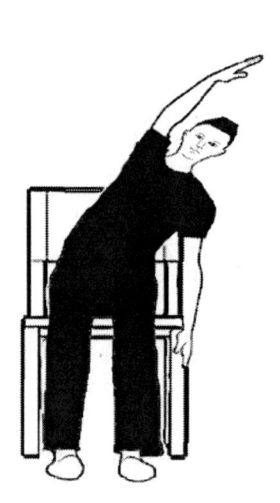

Checklist
- ✓ Stand or sit up straight
- ✓ Do this stretch once in each direction
- ✓ Do not lean forward, twist, or let the top arm come forward
- ✓ Hold the stretch for five to ten deep belly breaths
- ✓ Use diaphragmatic breathing through the nose as much as possible
- ✓ When standing keep the knees slightly bent
- ✓ Do not exercise to the point of strain or discomfort

Arm Circles

This movement will help to loosen the shoulders. Check your posture before you begin. Shoulders should be back and down and over the hips. Knees should remain slightly bent. Tuck the chin in and think about pushing the crown of the head up to the ceiling without lifting your chin. The abdominal muscles are lightly pulled in, but not so much as to restrict your breathing.

Lift both arms out to the side, shoulder height if you can. Turn the palms so they face up to the ceiling. Push the hands out to both sides to lengthen the arms and try to straighten the elbows without locking them. Move the hands back as far as you can to open the chest, but not so far as to cause discomfort in your shoulders. Holding here, make five small arm circles *backwards*. Focus on going backwards in order to open the chest and shoulders. Circling forwards can cause rounding of the shoulders, the exact postural habit that we are trying to change. Then relax your arms down by your sides. Repeat three to five more times.

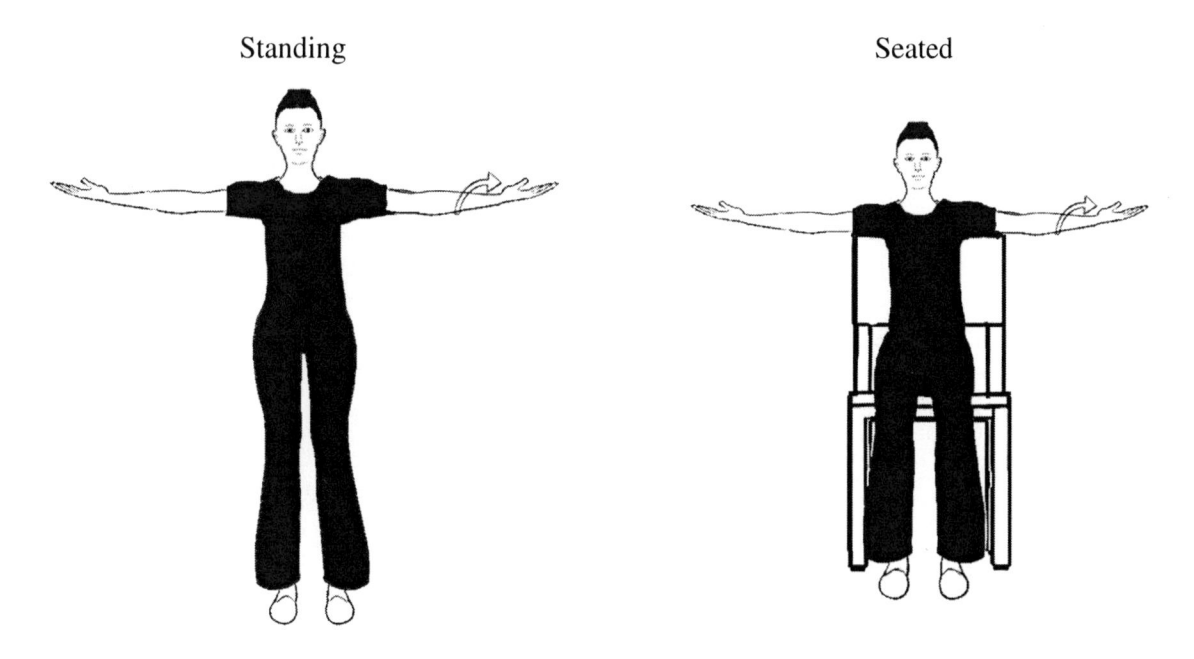

Standing   Seated

Checklist
- ✓ Stand or sit up straight
- ✓ Use diaphragmatic breathing through the nose as much as possible
- ✓ Keep the knees slightly bent
- ✓ Make sure you circle the arms backwards, not forwards
- ✓ Stretch your arms out to the sides and bring them back as far as you can to open the chest
- ✓ Do not exercise to the point of strain or discomfort

Squats

This movement strengthens the muscles in the front top of the thigh, and helps to loosen the knee joints. Check your posture before you begin. Shoulders should be back and down and over the hips. Knees should remain slightly bent. Tuck the chin in and think about pushing the crown of the head up to the ceiling without lifting your chin. The abdominal muscles are lightly pulled in, but not so much as to restrict your breathing.

Have a chair behind you. Bring your arms up to chest height with the palms facing the floor. Allow the natural curve in the low back to remain throughout this movement. Bend your knees and reach your buttocks back as if you were going to sit in the chair. If able, lower the buttocks until you come into contact with the chair, but try not to sit all the way. If you can not go that far, just go as far as you are able.

If your knees are sensitive, use caution with this movement. Only go as low as you can without causing pain in the knees. Another way to help reduce knee discomfort is to widen your stance.

You will find that as your legs become stronger you will be able to go lower without knee pain or losing your balance. Keep the weight forward and in your toes. This helps balance the body and prevents you from falling backwards.

Move *gently and slowly*, counting *one-one thousand, two-one thousand, three-one thousand, four-one thousand* to get into the squat, and use the same count to come up out of the squat. Inhale as you lower down and exhale as you stand up. As you come to standing press into your heels to help engage the leg muscles. Make sure you do not lock the knees or push the hips forward when you come to standing. Repeat eight to twelve times.

Standing

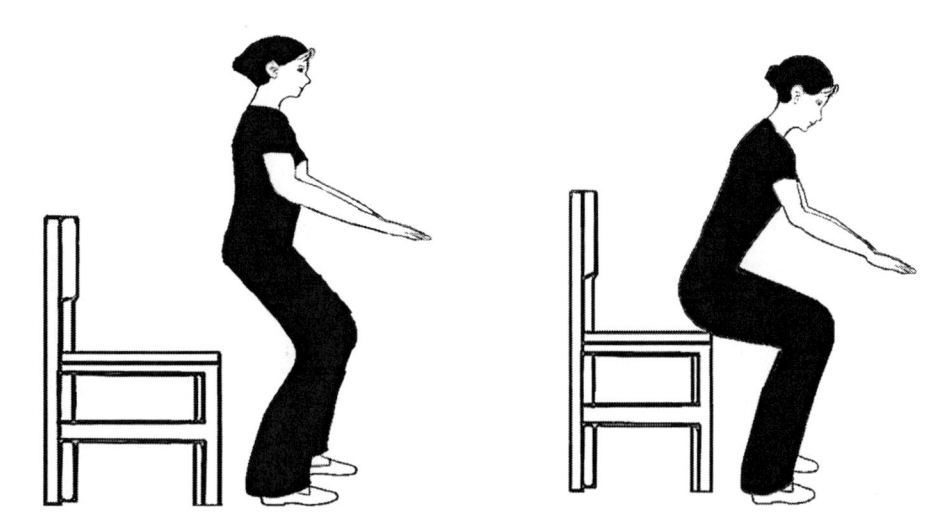

Standing with assistance

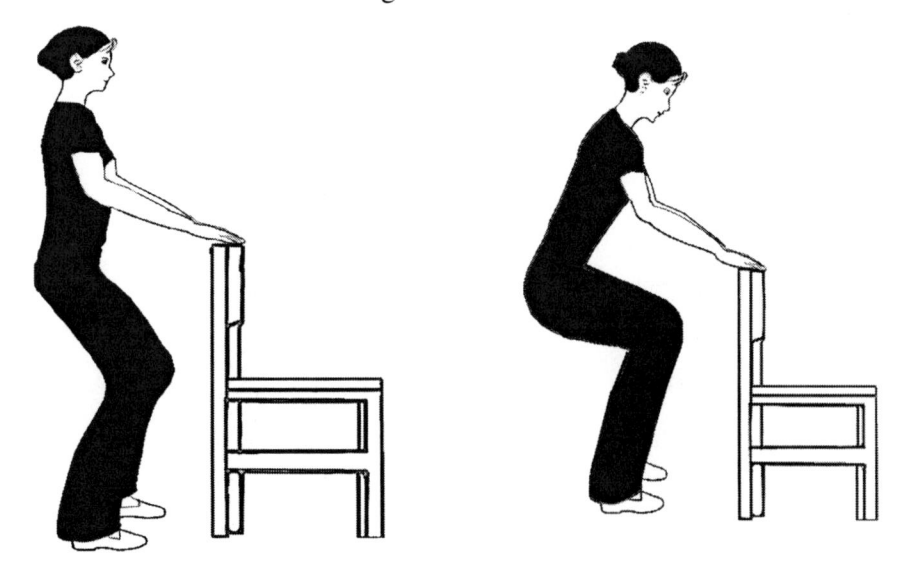

Checklist
- ✓ Stand up straight
- ✓ Move slowly using a "four thousand count" for each movement
- ✓ Use diaphragmatic breathing through the nose as much as possible
- ✓ Keep the natural arch in the low back
- ✓ Keep your weight forward and in your toes
- ✓ Do not exercise to the point of strain or discomfort

Overhead Stretch

This movement helps to loosen the shoulders and open the chest. Check your posture before you begin. Shoulders should be back and down and over the hips. Knees should remain slightly bent. Tuck the chin in and think about pushing the crown of the head up to the ceiling without lifting your chin. The abdominal muscles are lightly pulled in, but not so much as to restrict your breathing.

Lift your arms up overhead clasping the fingers if possible. If you can not go that far just reach your arms up. Turn your hands so your palms face the ceiling. Press your palms up to the ceiling, try to straighten your elbows, but do not lock them. Bring the arms back towards your ears as far as you can, without hurting your shoulders. Hold for five to ten deep belly breaths. Each time you inhale try to stretch up further, draw the arms back and straighten the elbows. Each time you exhale relax the shoulders. Repeat five more times.

Standing   Seated

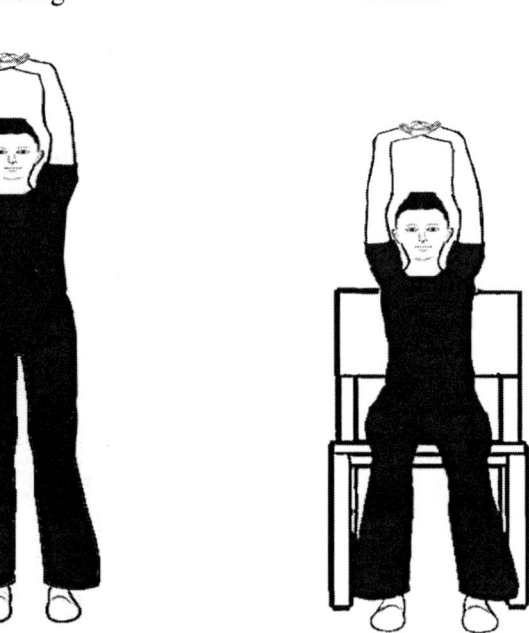

Checklist
- ✓ Stand or sit up straight
- ✓ Use diaphragmatic breathing through the nose as much as possible
- ✓ Keep the knees slightly bent when standing
- ✓ Do not exercise to the point of strain or discomfort

Chest Stretch

This movement will help to open the chest and the shoulders and correct a forward rounded posture. This stretch is good after working at a desk or computer for some time.

Check your posture before you begin. Shoulders should be back and down and over the hips. Knees should remain slightly bent. Tuck the chin in and think about pushing the crown of the head up to the ceiling without lifting your chin. The abdominal muscles are lightly pulled in, but not so much as to restrict your breathing.

If you can, clasp your hands behind your back. If you are unable to clasp your hands, just reach back. Keep your knees slightly bent. Draw your shoulder blades together and lift your hands away from your body as far as you can without hurting your shoulders. Be careful to not lean forward as you lift your hands. Your shoulders should stay over your hips. Move *gently and slowly,* counting *one-one thousand, two-one thousand, three-one thousand, four-one thousand* to lift your arms, and use the same count to lower the arms down. Repeat eight to twelve times.

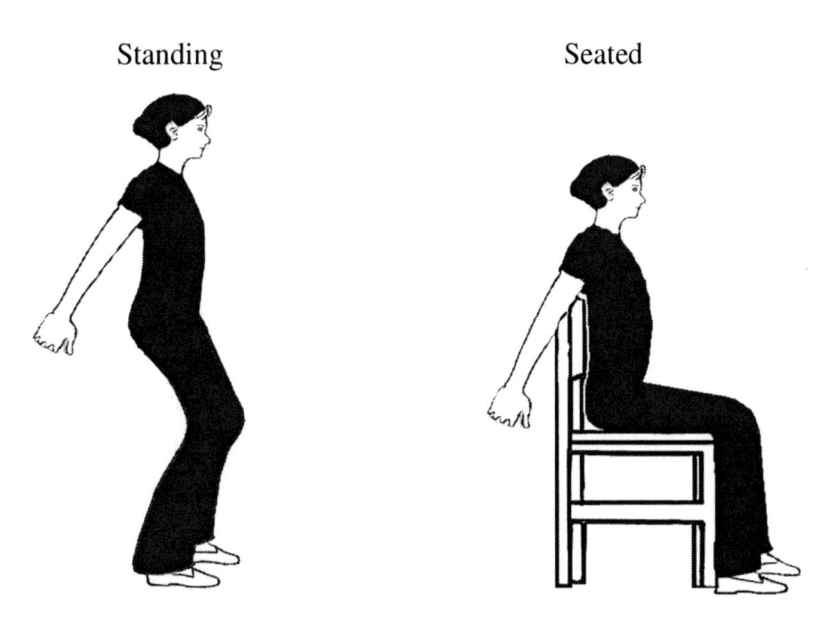

Standing   Seated

Checklist
- ✓ Stand or sit up straight
- ✓ Use diaphragmatic breathing through the nose as much as possible
- ✓ Keep the knees slightly bent when standing
- ✓ Do not lean forward as you lift the arms
- ✓ Do not exercise to the point of strain or discomfort

Summary

This completes the warm-up segment, which usually takes between ten to twenty minutes to complete. If you are new to exercising, or having a day when you are not feeling well, these range of motion exercises may be a good place to start.

Also, stretching is essential for those with Parkinson's Disease. Regular stretching promotes flexibility and can counteract the rigidity and stiffness brought on by PD. Good flexibility is necessary for all daily functional activities. If you become sedentary you may find that your muscles become tighter and your range of motion will become more and more limited. When your flexibility is reduced tasks such as walking, reaching, dressing, and bathing become more difficult.

Another concern is that as the muscles in your trunk become tighter you will start to develop a rounded back and hunched posture. This posture brings your body out of balance and can increase your chances of a fall and it also decreases your lung capacity.

The range of motion exercises in this chapter provide a total body stretching routine to help you maintain good posture and improve your flexibility.

"My daughter was planning her wedding and I wanted to give her away but my balance and stiff movements made it necessary to use a walker or cane. However, after just a couple of months of doing these range of motion exercises everyday, my flexibility improved. I was able to walk my daughter down the isle with pride, and no walker!"
- L.S. Massachusetts.

Chapter Three
Aerobic Exercise

"You must do the things you think you cannot do."

Eleanor Roosevelt

One component of an exercise regimen is aerobic or cardiovascular exercise. This type of exercise includes any activity which is sustained and raises the heart and breathing rate. The purpose of aerobic exercise is to strengthen the heart and lungs, train the body to utilize oxygen more efficiently, and help maintain a healthy weight and blood pressure.

Examples of aerobic exercise include:
- Walking
- Biking
- Aerobic dancing
- Swimming

Regular aerobic exercise can help:
- Take off excess weight and help you maintain a healthy weight
- Strengthen the heart and lungs
- Improve stamina and endurance
- Reduce stress
- Improve mood and combat depression
- Help control high blood pressure and high cholesterol

Getting Started with Aerobic Exercise

How Often Should You Do Aerobic or Cardiovascular Exercise?

Thirty minutes of aerobic exercise at least three times per week is recommended. Five days per week is better, and some aerobic activity everyday is optimal. If you have not been exercising regularly, this would be too much to start with. If you are just beginning to exercise either for the first time, or after being away from it for a while, try for five to ten minutes two to three times per week. Then, each week try to add one to two minutes until you can comfortably do fifteen minutes three times per week. From there keep adding more and more time slowly, and eventually add additional days. A common mistake made by many is to start off too vigorously. This leads to muscle soreness and fatigue, making it difficult to keep exercising. Starting slowly and increasing gradually, allows the body to adapt to the exercise. While one can expect to feel some stiffness at the start, your routine should not cause pain or discomfort to the point where it restricts you from doing daily activities.

How Hard Should You Workout?

The goal of aerobic exercise is to raise the heart and breathing rate to a point where you will benefit from the routine. During aerobic classes it is commonly recommended to take your pulse (or your heart rate) during the exercise session, with a goal of sustaining it at a level equal to sixty to eighty percent of your heart's maximum ability. However, many medications can interfere with your heart rate. For example some heart medications work to keep your heart rate lower. When you start exercising the medication will continue to try to lower your heart rate. This means you may be working very hard, but your medication is working to keep lowering your heart rate. If you continue to try to increase your heart rate to sixty to eighty percent, you may be putting yourself at risk for injury. In other words, taking your heart rate may not be providing you with an accurate picture of how hard you are actually working. Another concern with taking your heart rate is that many people have a hard time locating their pulse. This can often cause people to stop exercising while they try to find their pulse. This causes the heart rate to drop, which interferes with keeping the exercise at a steady pace. Given this, many people choose to use a scale known as the Rating of Perceived Exertion. This scale assigns a number to describe how hard you feel you are working. It is a self-rating technique you can do periodically during your routine to judge if you are working at the right level to gain benefits. At periods throughout your routine take a moment to use the following scale to rate how you are feeling.

The Rating of Perceived Exertion scale is as follows:

1	No effort, resting
2	Very, Very Light
3	Very Light
4	Fairly Light
5	Moderate
6	Somewhat Hard
7	Hard
8	Very Hard
9	Very, Very Hard
10	Maximum Effort/Exhaustion

For your aerobic program, you should gradually work up to a level between five and seven. Working at a level between one and four will not be vigorous enough to get the full benefit from your routine. Working above level seven may lead to soreness, injury and fatigue.

Another way to test how hard you are working is the talk test. While exercising you should not be so out of breath that you can not even answer a yes or no question. If you are gasping for breath just to say a few words you are working too hard. If on the other hand you are able to carry on a full conversation with no trouble, you are not exercising hard enough!

How to deal with freezing

One issue for those with Parkinson's disease is trouble with "freezing" or as my students refer to it, "being stuck." This occurs when the body is having trouble initiating movement. This can make aerobic activities challenging. Below are some tips that help my students.

- Try to quickly lift up the toes of both feet or swing both arms up to shoulder height. This may jolt the body into moving.
- Count or speak out loud, saying '*one, two, three, four*' or "*step, step, step.*"
Speaking out loud creates a rhythm that can get the body going again.
- Sing or hum an easy song you know well. This also creates a rhythm for the body to follow.
- Carry a small metronome to provide a constant source of rhythm.
- Use music for your aerobic routine. It will provide a beat for the body to follow.

Not all of these techniques work for everyone all of the time. Experiment with the different approaches until you find one or two that help you to start moving again.

How to find the right music

Using music for the aerobic component also helps to ensure that you are working at a good pace in order to raise your heart rate high enough to get benefits. It also can make the time go by faster. Using music is also a good way to time your routine. However long you are aiming to exercise - five minutes, ten minutes, or a longer amount of time - try making a tape or CD that plays the same amount of time you want your routine to be. In my classes, I use music that is approximately 120 beats per minute.

To determine the beats per minute of a song do the following:

- Get a stopwatch or watch with a second hand.
- Play the music you wish to use.
- Tap to the beat of the song with your hand or foot.
- Count how many times you tap in a fifteen second period.
- You should count about thirty beats. (30 times four is 120. We times the thirty beats by four, as there are four fifteen second periods per minute).
- If you find that this speed of music too fast to keep up with, start with slower music and gradually work up to music that is 120 beats per minute.

Why You Need to Exercise Your Heart

The cardiovascular system is made up of the heart, blood, and blood vessels. The circulatory system is your body's delivery system. Blood leaving the heart delivers oxygen and nutrients to the body. On the way back to the heart, the blood picks up and carries away waste products.

The Heart Muscle

The heart is a very important muscle of the body. In an average lifetime the heart beats more than two and a half billion times and is often described as a pump. It pumps blood around your body supplying the cells with nutrients and removing waste. An adult's heart pumps nearly 4000 gallons of blood each day. It contracts on average between sixty to eighty times a minute, more if you are exercising or exerting yourself. This number is known as your "heart rate."

The heart contains four chambers, and is shaped and sized roughly like a man's fist. The top two chambers are called the atria and the bottom two chambers are called the ventricles.

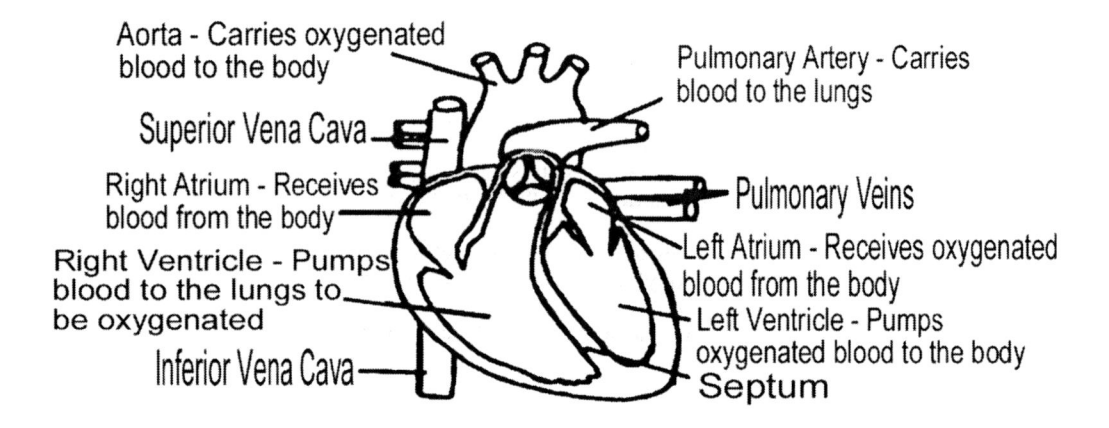

- Aorta - Carries oxygenated blood to the body
- Pulmonary Artery - Carries blood to the lungs
- Superior Vena Cava
- Right Atrium - Receives blood from the body
- Pulmonary Veins
- Right Ventricle - Pumps blood to the lungs to be oxygenated
- Left Atrium - Receives oxygenated blood from the body
- Inferior Vena Cava
- Left Ventricle - Pumps oxygenated blood to the body
- Septum

Exercise and your Heart

Regular aerobic exercise is the best method of keeping the heart muscle strong and healthy as it places specific demands on the body. During aerobic exercise the muscles demand more oxygen-rich blood and give off more carbon dioxide and other waste. To accomplish this the heart must beat faster, and pump more blood with each beat to meet these demands. This means that your heart rate and blood pressure must increase in order to supply the working muscles with an increased need for blood and oxygen.

The effects of regular exercise will depend on the type, duration, frequency and intensity of training. Since the heart muscle must work harder to accommodate the increased needs during exercise, the heart muscle will become stronger and more efficient. When you give your heart a workout on a regular basis it will become better at its main job, delivering blood and oxygen to all parts of your body. When you follow a program of regular aerobic exercise, over time your heart grows stronger and can meet the muscles' demands both during exercise and daily activities with less effort.

Exercise and Blood Pressure

Blood pressure measures the pressure the blood exerts against the walls of the arteries. This pressure changes constantly according to the body's needs. In very general terms the systolic pressure measures the pressure exerted when your heart beats. The diastolic pressure measures the pressure when your heart relaxes. The average systolic blood pressure is 100 to 140 mmHg (mm of mercury). The average diastolic pressure is 60 to 85 mmHg. This determines the blood pressure, which is recorded as a fraction such as 120/80 mmHg. *Hypertension* (high blood pressure) is defined in an adult as a blood pressure greater than or equal to 140 mm Hg systolic pressure or greater than or equal to 90 mmHg diastolic pressure. As mentioned above, regular aerobic exercise makes your heart stronger. A stronger heart pumps more blood with less effort. This means there is less work for your heart to do, and therefore less force or pressure, that's exerted on your arteries. The less pressure on the arteries, the lower your blood pressure.

To review, regular aerobic exercise strengthens the heart and lowers blood pressure as it can:

- Make your resting heart rate slower – meaning your heart is not having to work as hard
- Increase the size of major coronary vessels, making it easier for the blood to flow to all regions of the heart - in other words there is more space and less resistance for the blood to flow through as it travels throughout the body
- Increase the amount of blood the heart pumps with every beat
- Increase the size and pumping ability of the heart - as with all of the muscles in the body, when the heart muscle is stressed through exercise it gets stronger
- Increase the number of capillaries in the body thereby aiding in the distribution of blood
- Lower blood pressure due to a stronger more efficient system
- Lead to a decrease in body fat and weight, so there is less area for the body to have to supply blood to

Regular aerobic exercise produces a more efficient system that recovers quicker. Oftentimes when you first begin to exercise you get out of breath quickly, and when you stop exercising it takes a while to catch your breath. However this improves with regular exercise. You will notice that after about four to eight weeks of regular aerobic exercise you will not get out of breath as quickly, and when you stop exercising your blood pressure, rate of breathing, and heart rate will recover to their pre-exercise levels more quickly then before. This means that your body is adapting to the exercise program and is becoming more efficient.

Why You Need To Exercise Your Lungs

You breathe with the help of your diaphragm and other muscles in your chest and abdomen. These muscles literally change the space and pressure inside the body to accommodate breathing. Your lungs are like a pair of balloons that expand when you inhale. When you inhale, your diaphragm drops down so the lung cavity can expand and take in air. When you exhale the muscles squeeze your rib cage, your diaphragm moves upwards, your lungs begin to collapse, and the air is pushed up and out of your body.

You breathe in about twenty times per minute. Every minute you inhale approximately thirteen pints of air. In the course of a day, approximately 8,000 to 9,000 liters of inhaled air meets 8,000 to 10,000 liters of blood pumped in by the heart through the pulmonary artery (see pg. 80). The air you inhale passes through the nasal passages which filter, heat, and moisten the air before it flows into the back of the throat. The air then flows down through the trachea (windpipe) and eventually into the lungs. Inside each of your lungs are millions of tiny sacs called alveoli. Here, the red blood cells interact with these sacs to trade in the old carbon dioxide that your body's cells have made, for some new oxygen you have just breathed in.

The "new" oxygen passes through the walls of each alveoli into the tiny capillaries that surround them and enters the blood, where it is carried by red blood cells to the heart. The heart then sends the oxygen-rich blood through arteries and capillaries to all the cells in the body.

Veins then carry the oxygen-depleted blood back to the heart and then onto the lungs. Here, the carbon dioxide and waste picked up by the alveoli travels through the lungs, back up your windpipe and it is expelled with every exhale.

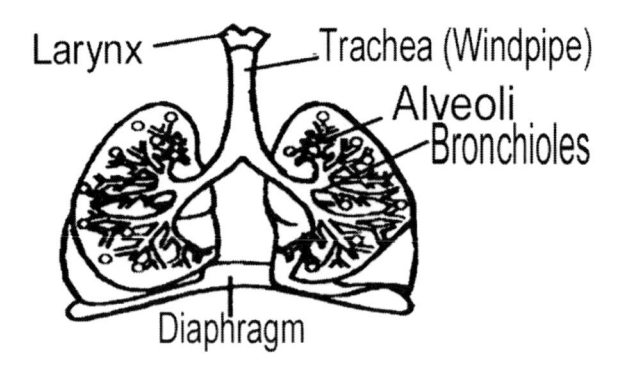

Exercise and Your Respiratory System

Aerobic exercise places demands on the system which results in a stronger respiratory system, making it more efficient at delivering and processing oxygen in the body. *Cardiorespiratory endurance* (the health of our heart and lungs) refers to the body's ability to sustain prolonged activity. The endurance of this system can be tested by measuring the highest rate of oxygen consumption attainable during maximal exertion. This level of maximal exertion is known as your "V02 max." When you reach this level your body can no longer deliver oxygen as quickly as your muscles need to receive it. Thus you will not be able to continue the activity you were doing for much longer. Regular aerobic activity has been shown to increase this level, allowing you to perform activities for longer periods at a higher intensity.

Regular aerobic exercise brings about other changes in the body's respiratory system enabling it to function more effectively. Regular aerobic exercise forces the lungs to work harder and faster to deliver the needed oxygen, which strengthens and conditions them. Exercise is good for every part of your body, especially your lungs and heart. When you take part in regular exercise your lungs require more air to give your cells the extra oxygen they need. As you breathe more deeply and take in more air, your lungs become stronger and more efficient at supplying your body with the air it needs for exercise and everyday activities. Below are some of the benefits of regular aerobic exercise.

- Makes your respiratory system stronger and more efficient
- Increases the amount of air the lungs can breathe in and out during all activities
- Your breathing rate becomes slower even at rest, meaning your lungs are not having to work as hard
- Improves lung capacity and strengthens the diaphragm muscle. This is crucial for those with Parkinson's disease. An increase in lung capacity means that you do not get out of breath as quickly during all types of activity (such as climbing stairs and walking uphill), and it helps with the ability to speak louder and project your voice.
- Decreases fatigue. After approximately six to eight weeks of regular aerobic exercise you may find that you are less tired during exercise and everyday activities.
- Induces sleep. Many of my class participants who do regular aerobic exercise notice that they sleep better at night.
- Increases your tolerance for exercise. You will find you can exercise longer and at a harder pace then when you started.

The Aerobic Exercises

The following movements are some of the ones I use in my program. They move the body in a variety of directions to fully work the joints and muscles. Challenging the body to travel in different directions such as forward, backwards, and sideways also helps to improve balance. Because there are many other ways to move the body, you may wish to vary this routine with other movements you know. Aerobic exercise can be done standing, standing and holding onto a chair or counter for support, or while seated. *Try to do as much as you can standing*. This will help to improve balance and provide weight bearing exercise to help strengthen the bones, as well as improving your cardiovascular health.

Experiment with the different variations to find the right option for you. You can do some of each. For example, if you are new to exercise or having a day when you are not feeling well, you may choose to do a few repetitions standing, and then a few repetitions seated. As with everything in this program explore different approaches to see what feels best. The movements will be shown one per page with instructions. The last page will list all the movements together and provides sample sequences so you can move through your routine more smoothly.

Before beginning aerobic exercise, make sure you warm-up by taking a short walk, or performing the warm-up exercises in chapter two. After completing aerobic activity, it is important to let the body cool down slowly by continuing with some type of gentle movement for another three to five minutes to let the heart and breathing rate slowly adjust back to their pre-exercise level.

My husband and I love to walk. After he developed Parkinson's it became more difficult for him. I found myself having to walk slower so we could stay together. Since he started taking the aerobics class, he has learned to focus on taking large steps and swinging his arms when he walks – I now have to work to keep up with him!   - P. W.   Massachusetts

Marching in Place

Standing
Alternately lift the feet off the floor and swing the arms.

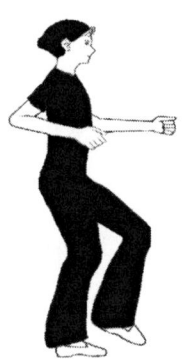

Standing with assistance
Do not lean on the chair; just a light fingertip grip. Let your legs support you.

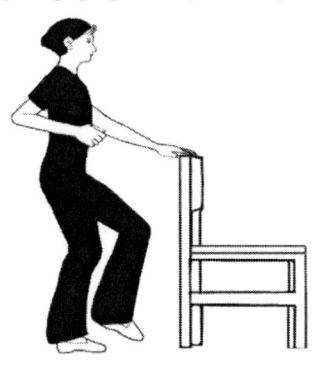

Seated
Sit up straight and away from the back of the chair as much as possible.

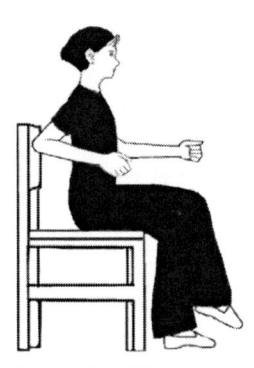

Checklist
- ✓ Stand or sit up straight and do as much as you can standing without holding on
- ✓ Swing your arms, using opposite arm to leg to help maintain balance
- ✓ Focus on picking the feet up so that they come completely off the floor
- ✓ Use the Rating of Perceived Exertion or talk test (pg. 78) to check if you are exercising at the right level
- ✓ Breathe

Alternate Straight Leg Kicks

Standing

Alternately kick forward with a straight leg keeping your balance and your back straight. Swing the opposite arm to leg.

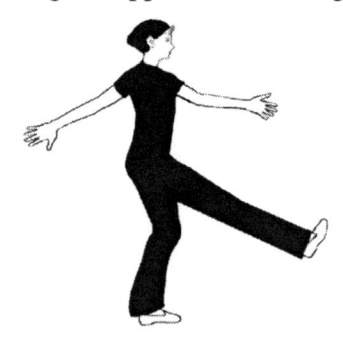

Standing with assistance

Do not lean on the chair; just a light fingertip grip. Let your legs support you.

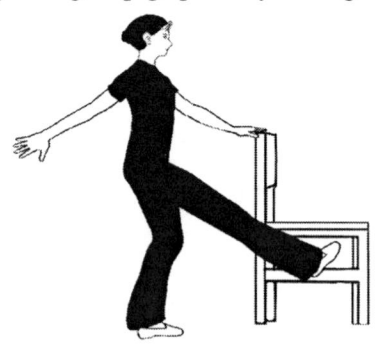

Seated

Sit up straight and away from the back of the chair as much as possible.

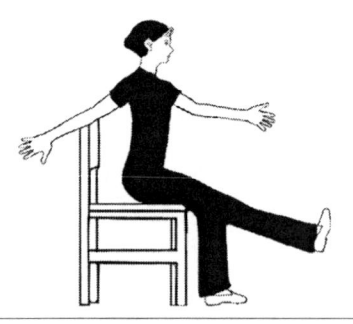

Checklist
- ✓ Stand or sit up straight and do as much as you can standing without holding on
- ✓ Swing your arms, using opposite arm to leg to help maintain balance
- ✓ Focus on keeping the knee straight
- ✓ Use the Rating of Perceived Exertion or talk test (pg. 78) to check if you are exercising at the right level
- ✓ Breathe

Stepping Side to Side
Standing

Stand with feet together.   Step out to the right.   Bring the left foot to the right foot

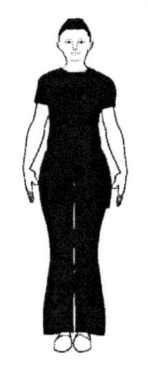

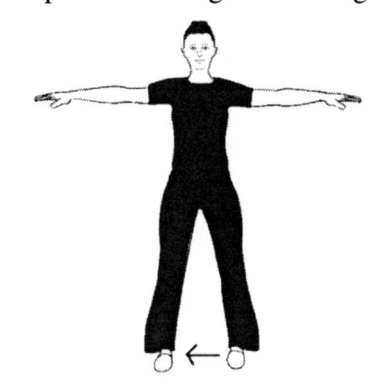

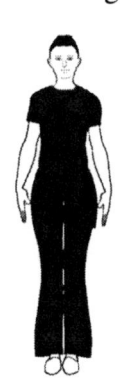

Take as wide of a step as possible.

Stand with feet together.   Step out to the left.   Bring the right foot to the left foot

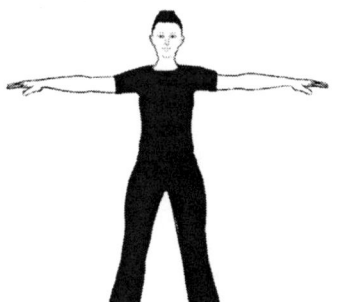

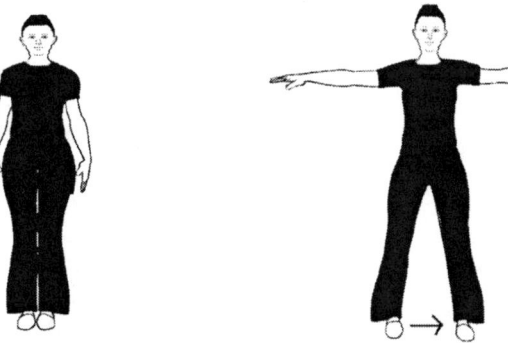

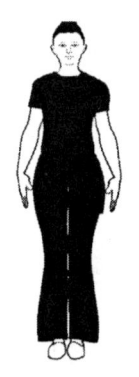

Continue stepping from right to left. Try to swing the arms up to shoulder height.

Standing with assistance

Do not lean on the chair; try to keep just a light fingertip grip. Let your legs work to support you. Step out to the right and bring the left foot to the right. Take as wide of a step as possible.

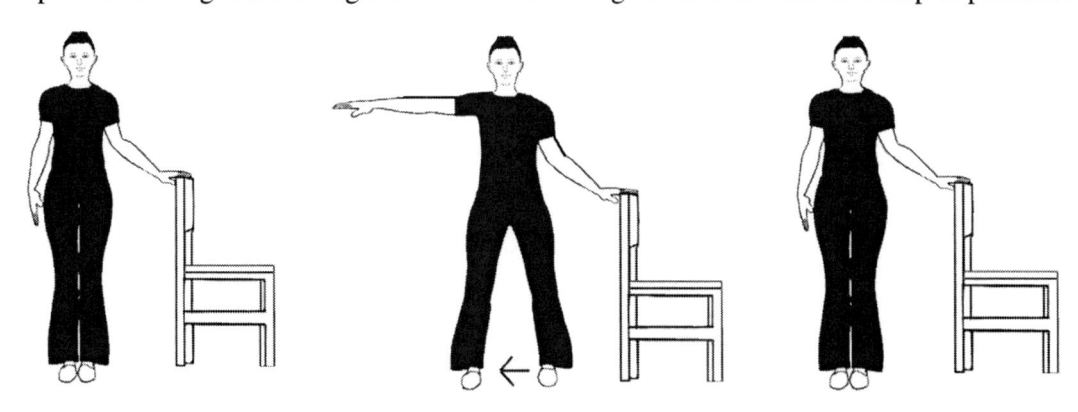

Step out to the left and bring the right foot to the left.

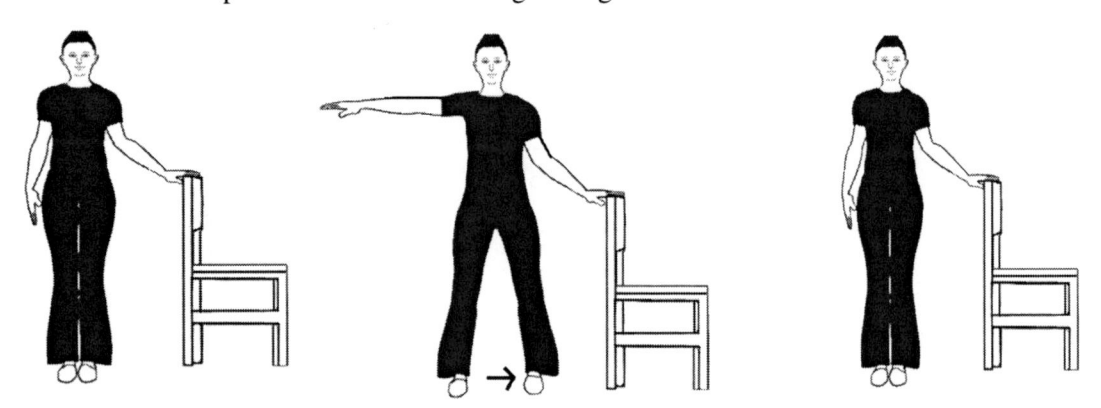

Continue stepping from right to left. Swing the free arm up to shoulder height.

Seated
Sit up straight and away from the back of the chair as much as possible.
Step out to the right and bring the left foot to the right. Take as wide of a step as possible.

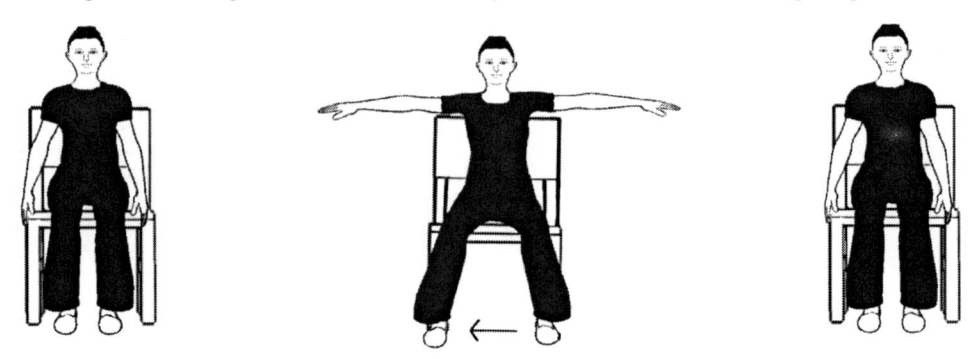

Step out to the left and bring the right foot to the left.
Continue stepping from right to left. Try to swing the arms up to shoulder height.

Checklist
- ✓ Stand or sit up straight try to do as much as you can standing without holding on
- ✓ Swing your arms up to shoulder height
- ✓ Focus on taking as wide of a step as you can
- ✓ Use the Rating of Perceived Exertion or talk test (pg. 78) to check if you are exercising at the right level
- ✓ Breathe

Alternate Knee Lifts

Standing

Alternately lift your knees as high as you can while keeping your balance and your back straight. Swing the opposite arm to leg.

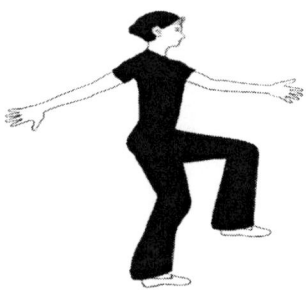

Standing with assistance

Do not lean on the chair; just use a light fingertip grip. Let your legs support you.

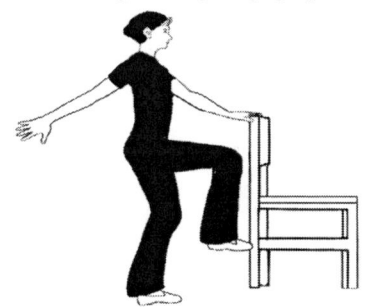

Seated

Sit up straight and away from the back of the chair as much as possible.

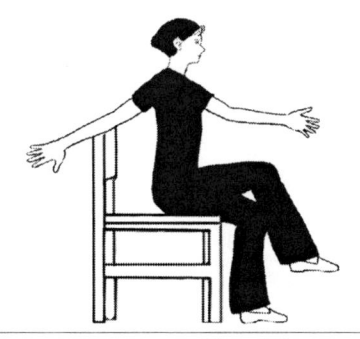

Checklist
- ✓ Stand or sit up straight and do as much as you can standing without holding on
- ✓ Swing your arms, using opposite arm to leg
- ✓ Focus on bringing the knee up to waist high if you can
- ✓ Use the Rating of Perceived Exertion or talk test (pg. 78) to check if you are exercising at the right level
- ✓ Breathe

Alternate Heel Curls Back

Standing

Alternately lift your heels to the back as high as you can, keeping your balance and your back straight. Swing the opposite arm forward.

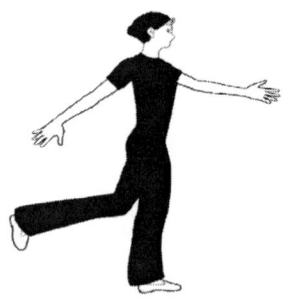

Standing with assistance

Do not lean on the chair; keep a light fingertip grip. Let your legs support you.

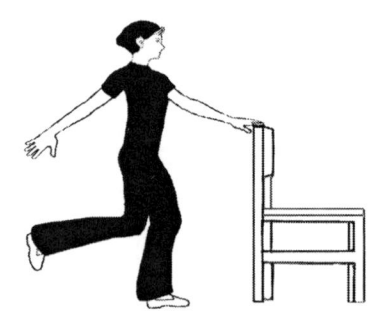

Seated

Sit up straight and away from the back of the chair as much as possible.

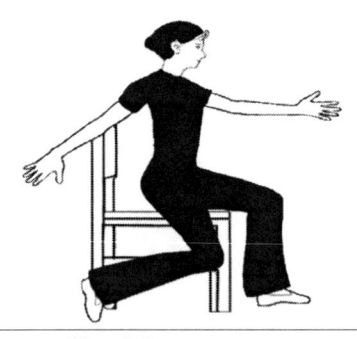

Checklist

- ✓ Stand or sit up straight and do as much as you can standing without holding on
- ✓ Swing your arms, using opposite arm to leg
- ✓ Focus on bringing the heel up to the back as high as you can
- ✓ Use the Rating of Perceived Exertion or talk test (pg. 78) to check if you are exercising at the right level
- ✓ Breathe

Side Toe Tap

Standing

Reach the right toe out to the side, as the arms lift up. Do not put any weight on the toe. Keep your weight in the left leg. Bring the right leg back to the center.

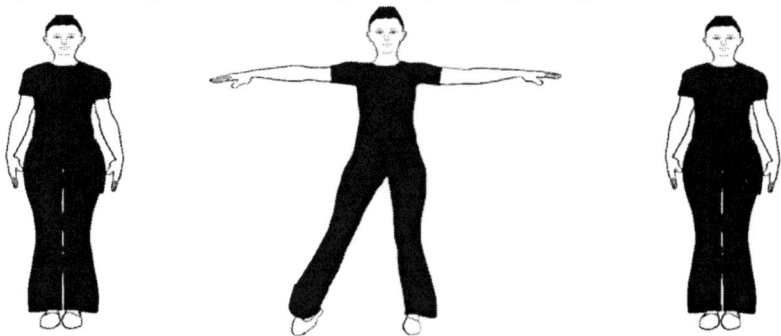

Reach the left toe out to the side, as the arms lift up. Do not put any weight on the toe. Keep your weight in the right leg. Bring the left leg back to the center. Continue alternating from side to side.

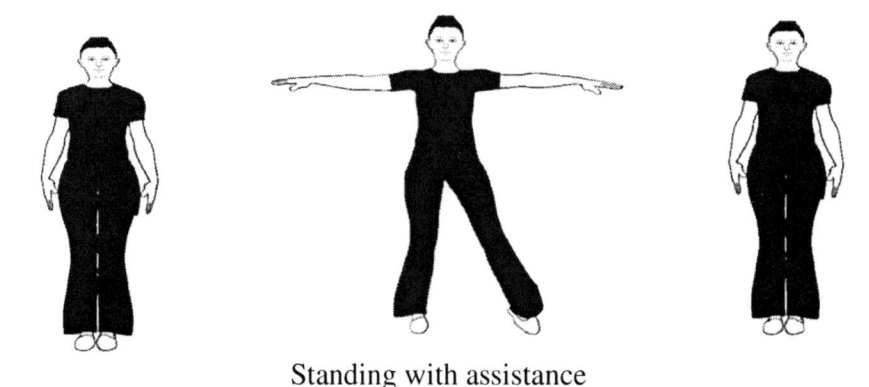

Standing with assistance

Do not lean on the chair; just use a light fingertip grip. Let your legs support you.

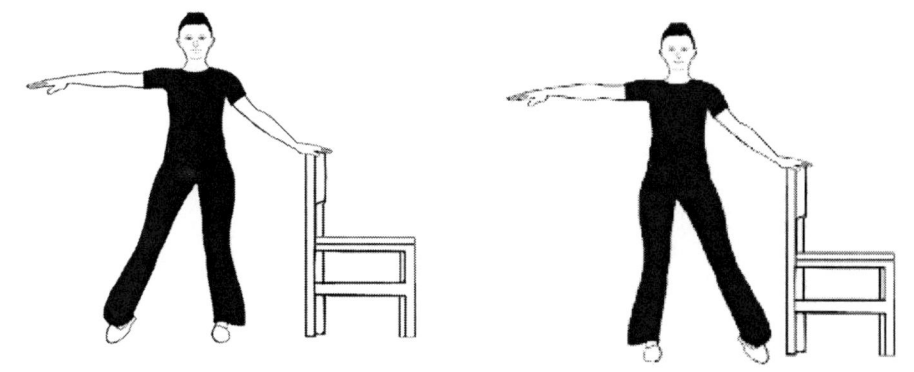

Continue alternating from side to side.

Seated

Sit up straight and away from the back of the chair as much as possible.

Continue alternating from side to side.

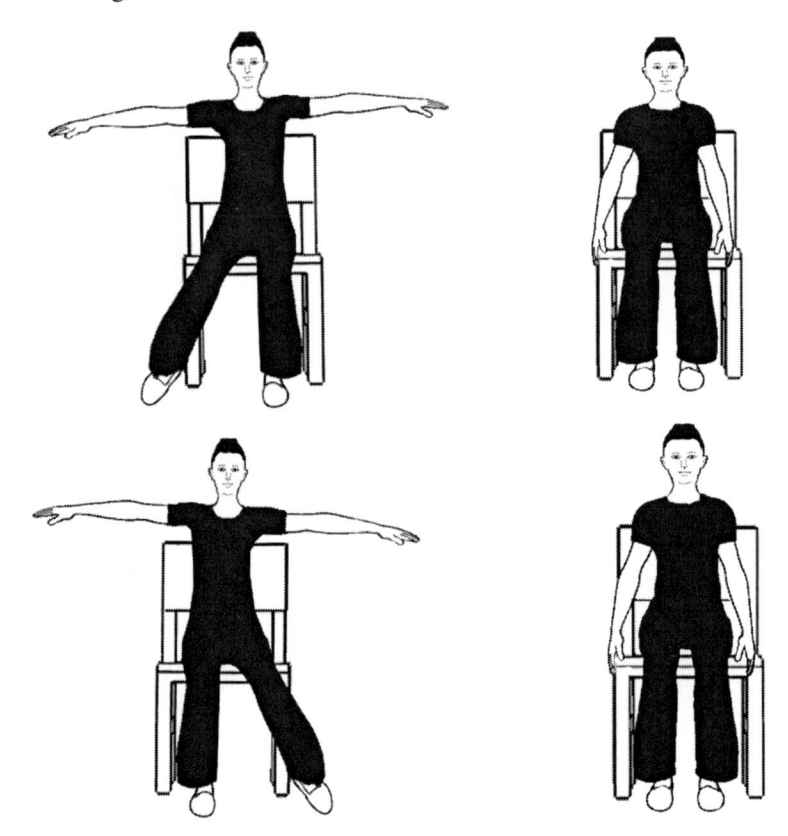

Checklist
- ✓ Stand or sit up straight and do as much as you can standing without holding on
- ✓ Swing your arms, trying to bring them shoulder height
- ✓ Reach the toe directly out to the side as far as you can without putting any weight on it
- ✓ Face forward through this movement. Do not twist the back or knees
- ✓ Use the Rating of Perceived Exertion or talk test (pg. 78) to check if you are exercising at the right level
- ✓ Breathe

Alternate Forward Heel Taps

Standing

Flex the foot and tap just the heel of the foot on the ground in front of you. Do not place the whole foot on the floor, or put any weight on the front foot. Alternately tap the heels in front. Swing the opposite arm to foot.

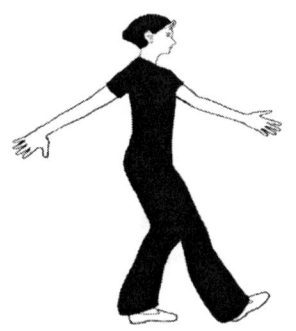

Standing with assistance

Do not lean on the chair; just use a light fingertip grip. Let your legs support you.

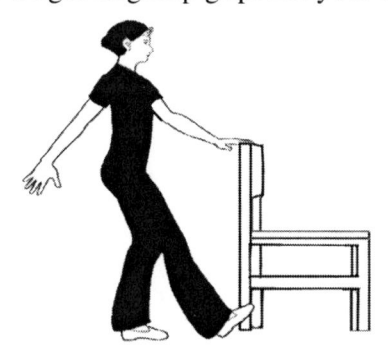

Seated

Sit up straight and away from the back of the chair as much as possible.

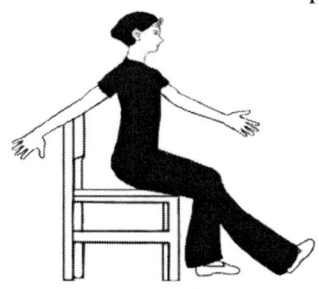

Checklist
- ✓ Stand or sit up straight and do as much as you can standing without holding on
- ✓ Swing your arms, using opposite arm to leg to help maintain balance
- ✓ Focus on touching just the heel on the floor and keeping your weight in your back leg
- ✓ Use the Rating of Perceived Exertion (pg. 78) to check if you are exercising at the right level
- ✓ Breathe

Putting It All Together

The following provides some sample routines to help you put together an aerobic workout based on the movements shown in this chapter. There are four different sample routines based on how long you want to exercise for. As mentioned earlier in this chapter if you have not been exercising regularly try starting with the three or seven minute workout and gradually as you feel able try to do a longer routine. These samples can also be helpful if you find that you only have a few minutes.

The most important thing to remember about using exercise to manage your symptoms is that you need to exercise on a regular basis. While it is optimal to do aerobic exercise for thirty minutes three to five times per week you may find that some days you do not have time or feel able to do that much. Instead of skipping your routine all together try doing a shorter workout so you keep yourself in the rhythm of regular exercise. Sometimes once you get started you will get the energy you need to do more.

Sample Routines

The 3 1/2 Minute Workout.
1. March in Place …. 30 seconds
2. Alternate Straight Leg Kicks …. 30 seconds
3. Stepping Side to Side…. 30 seconds
4. Alternate Knee Lifts…. 30 seconds
5. Alternate Heel Curls Back…. 30 seconds
6. Side Toe Tap…………. 30 seconds
7. Alternate Forward Heel Taps…. 30 seconds

The 7 Minute Workout
1. March in Place …. 60 seconds
2. Alternate Straight Leg Kicks …. 60 seconds
3. Stepping Side to Side…. 60 seconds
4. Alternate Knee Lifts…. 60 seconds
5. Alternate Heel Curls Back…. 60 seconds
6. Side Toe Tap…. 60 seconds
7. Alternate Forward Heel Taps…. 60 seconds

The 10 Minute Workout.
1. March in Place …. 43 seconds
2. Alternate Straight Leg Kicks … 43 seconds
3. Stepping Side to Side…. 43 seconds
4. Alternate Knee Lifts…. 43 seconds
5. Alternate Heel Curls Back…. 43 seconds
6. Side Toe Tap…. 43 seconds
7. Alternate Forward Heel Taps…. 43 seconds
8. March in Place …. 43 seconds
9. Alternate Straight Leg Kicks … 43 seconds
10. Stepping Side to Side…. 43 seconds
11. Alternate Knee Lifts…. 43 seconds
12. Alternate Heel Curls Back…. 43 seconds
13. Side Toe Tap…. 43 seconds
14. Alternate Forward Heel Taps…. 43 seconds

The 14 Minute Workout.
1. March in Place …. 60 seconds
2. Alternate Straight Leg Kicks …. 60 seconds
3. Stepping Side to Side…. 60 seconds
4. Alternate Knee Lifts…. 60 seconds
5. Alternate Heel Curls Back…. 60 seconds
6. Side Toe Tap…. 60 seconds
7. Alternate Forward Heel Taps…. 60 seconds
8. March in Place …. 60 seconds
9. Alternate Straight Leg Kicks …. 60 seconds
10. Stepping Side to Side…. 60 seconds
11. Alternate Knee Lifts…. 60 seconds
12. Alternate Heel Curls Back…. 60 seconds
13. Side Toe Tap…. 60 seconds
14. Alternate Forward Heel Taps…. 60 seconds

Checklist
- ✓ Try creating your own sequence of movements and move around the room; march forward and back for 8, or when side stepping, travel 4 steps right then left, etc.
- ✓ Remember the object is to keep moving, and to keep the heart rate up
- ✓ Try incorporating your favorite music into your routine
- ✓ Start slowly and build up gradually so your body can adapt. Listen to your body to determine the appropriate level for each day
- ✓ Use the Rating of Perceived Exertion or talk test (pg. 78) to check if you are exercising at the right level
- ✓ Breathe

Summary

Regular aerobic exercise is important to keep your heart and lungs strong, to maintain a healthy weight, and to help manage your blood pressure, heart rate, and cholesterol levels. You should aim for at least fifteen minutes of aerobic exercise every day, and if possible thirty minutes on at least three to five days per week. It is best to alternate between different activities. This could include doing the aerobic exercises in this book three days per week, and then walk, swim, bike or take a dance class on the other days. Whatever activity you choose make it fast paced enough to increase your heart rate and breathing. Aerobic exercise means maintaining an elevated heart rate throughout the fifteen to thirty minute session. So in terms of aerobic exercise, activities like housework, gardening, or yoga and tai chi are not enough. Techniques such as yoga and tai chi help to manage other areas such as flexibility and balance and they are covered later in this book.

The next chapter will cover strength training. With aerobic exercise the goal is to move quickly and raise your heart rate. In contrast strength training movements are done slowly and with control while moving your body against resistance, such as weights. This strengthens your muscles and will help make everyday activities such as getting out of a chair and climbing stairs easier and it also helps in preventing falls.

Note:

For some it is tempting to walk while holding hand weights or wearing ankle weights. Many people do this thinking they are getting both an aerobic workout and a strength training workout at the same time. Unfortunately you are just setting yourself up for injury. If you are walking fast enough to get aerobic benefit, then you are not using the weights with control. When walking the motion of your arms and legs is repetitive (swinging forward and back) so you are not isolating specific muscles. Also when you swing the arms and legs with weights on you place a lot of unnecessary stress on the joints and can end up with shoulder, hip, knee or ankle injuries.

Anytime you use weights the movements should be slow, and done with control and targeted at a specific muscle. You need to do a resistance exercise for each of your major muscle groups and move your body through various motions. Doing so is not only a more efficient way to strengthen your muscles, but it is also a safe way to train and reduces the risk of injury. *Your aerobic session and your strength training session should be separate activities.*

Chapter Four
Strength Training

"Never be bullied into silence. Never allow yourself to be made a victim. Accept no one's definition of your life; define yourself."

Harvey Fierstein

Strength training or resistance training is another important component of an exercise program for those with Parkinson's disease. As the muscles become stronger, certain tasks such as standing, walking, rising from a chair, climbing stairs, and lifting objects becomes easier. Benefits of strength training include stronger muscles that can do bigger jobs (such as lifting heavier objects), muscles that will work longer before becoming exhausted, an increase in lean body mass (more muscle, less fat), an increase in metabolism meaning more calories burned even at rest, better bone mineral density (stronger bones), improvements in overall stability and balance, lower blood sugar levels, decrease in body fat, fewer body aches and less fatigue.

Getting Started with Strength Training

Strength training or resistance training simply means performing movements against some kind of resistance. Such resistance can be your own body weight, free weights such as hand and ankle weights, theraband or tubing, or machines typically found at gyms. When beginning a strength training routine, it is advisable to have the guidance of an instructor to make sure you are performing the movements correctly. Aside from this you can get a complete and beneficial strength training workout at home.

How Much Weight Should You Use

If you have access to hand and ankle weights, this book will show you how to use them. However, when beginning an exercise routine you should use light weights. You will find that you will be able to increase the weight fairly quickly in the beginning. Eventually you will find a weight which you will use for a while. If you do not have weights at home you can use common household items to start, and wait to buy weights when you are ready for more resistance. Instead of hand weights try using full soup cans or cylinder-shaped plastic containers filled with water or sand. Plastic shampoo, milk bottles, or laundry detergent containers work well. For ankle weights you can substitute with an old pair of socks filled with sand to the appropriate weight. These can and then be tied or fastened with Velcro around your ankles.

Strength Training Exercises
Squats or Wall Slides *Muscles Worked: Quadriceps (Front top of thigh)*
(Rectus femoris, vastus lateralis, vastus medialis, vastus intermedius)

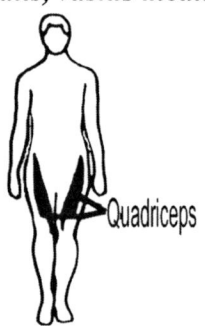

Squats

   Before starting, check your posture. Stand up straight, bring the hips under the shoulders, and think about pushing the crown of the head to the ceiling without lifting the chin.

   Have a chair behind you. Bring your arms up in front of you to chest height, with the palms facing the floor. Allow the natural curve in the low back to remain throughout this movement. Bend your knees and reach the buttocks back as if you were about to sit in a chair. If you are able, lower down until you come into contact with the chair, but do not actually sit. If you are not able to touch the chair, just go as far as you can. As your legs become stronger you will be able to go lower. Keep your weight forward and in your toes to avoid falling backwards. As you stand up, make sure you do not lock the knees and push the hips forward. Only stand up until there is a slight bend in the knees. Repeat for eight to twelve repetitions. If this movement bothers your knees, try taking a wider stance or do not go as low.

Standing

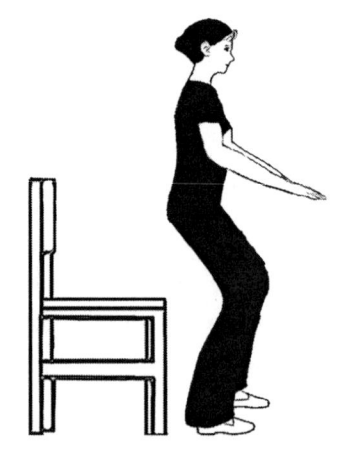

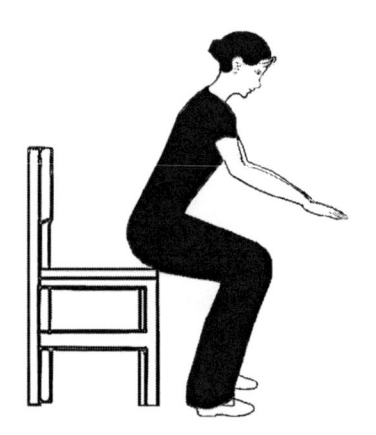

Against a Wall/Wall Slide

This exercise can also be done as a wall slide instead of a squat. Stand with the hips, back and shoulders against the wall. The feet are about one foot away from the wall. Slide down as far as you are able without hurting your knees. Keep your heels on the floor. The benefit of doing a wall slide is that it can help to correct a forward rounded posture. As you slide down, keep the back of your head, shoulder blades and buttocks against the wall. Make sure that you keep the head level and do not lift the chin in order to touch your head. Use the chin tuck exercise and just come as close to the wall as you can.

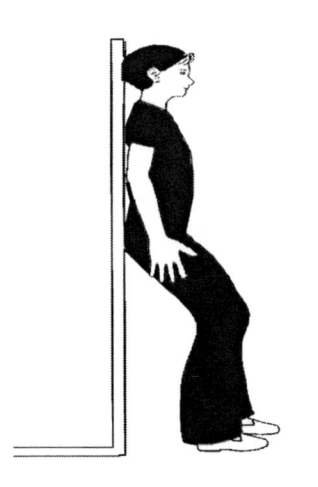

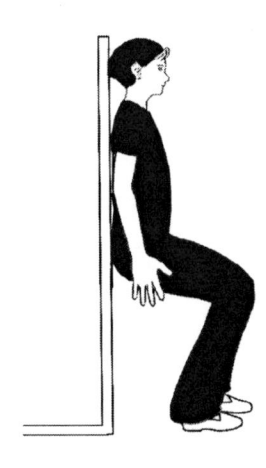

Checklist
✓ Stand or sit up straight.
✓ Move through your full range of motion, but do not lock the knee
✓ Move slowly using a "four thousand count" for each movement
✓ Keep the natural arch in the low back
✓ Use diaphragmatic breathing through the nose as much as possible
✓ Do not exercise to the point of strain or discomfort

Leg Extensions *Muscles Worked: Quadriceps (Front top of thigh)*
(Rectus femoris, vastus lateralis, vastus medialis, vastus intermedius)

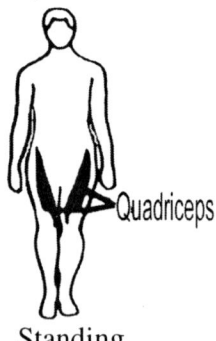

Standing

Before starting, check your posture. Stand up straight, bring the hips under the shoulders, and think about pushing the crown of the head to the ceiling without lifting the chin. Do eight to twelve repetitions with the right leg, then eight to twelve repetitions with the left leg.

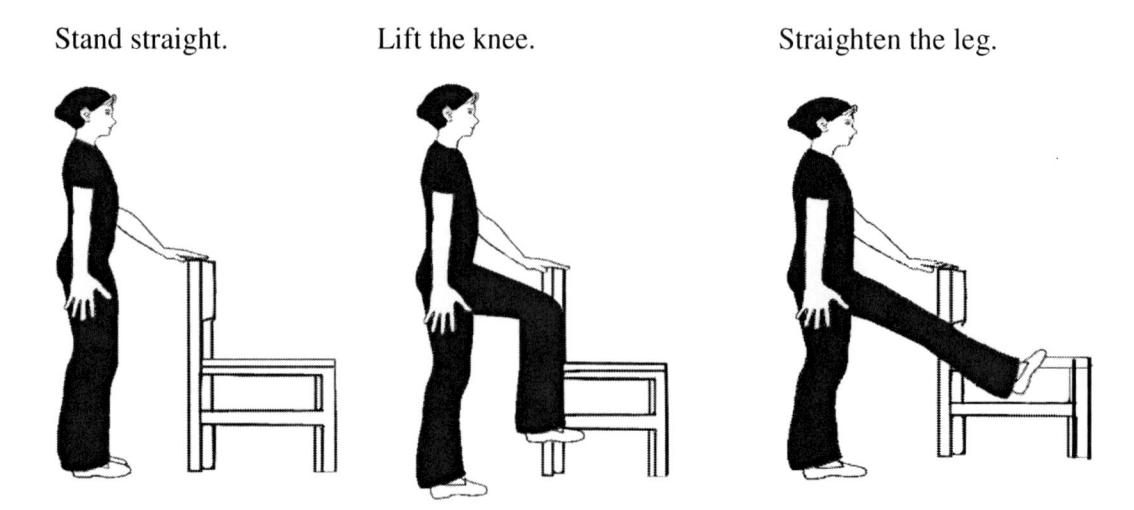

Stand straight.

Lift the knee.

Straighten the leg.

Bend the knee.

Put the foot down.

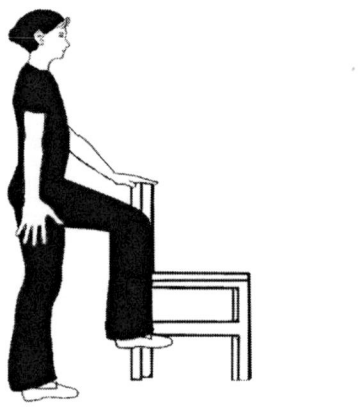

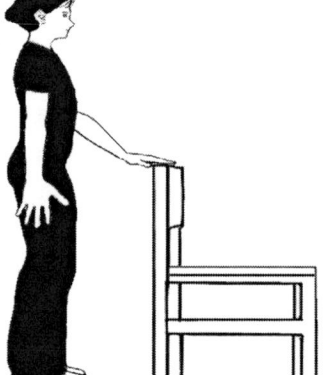

Seated

Sit up straight, away from the back of the chair if possible. If you need to sit back, sit all the way back to avoid slouching.

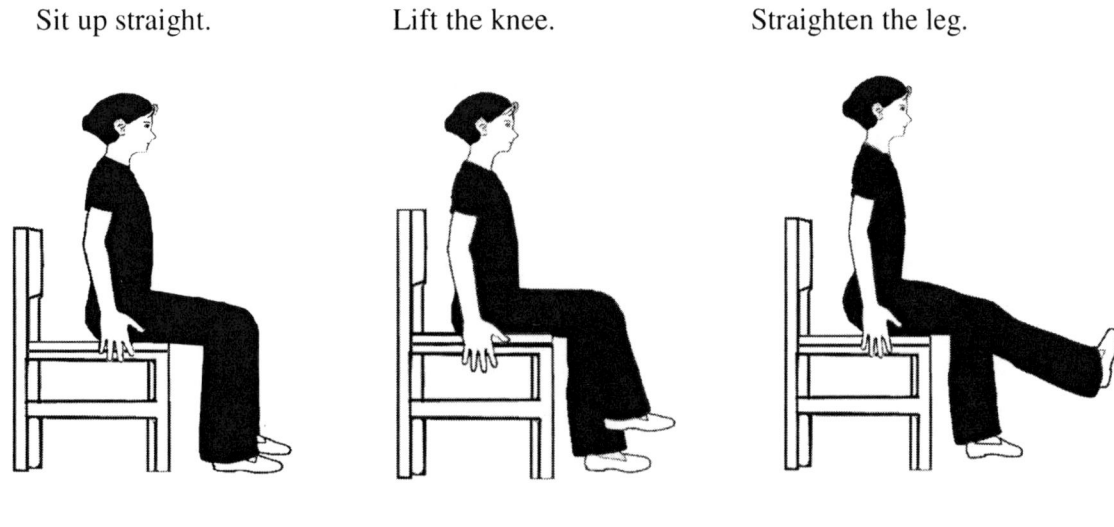

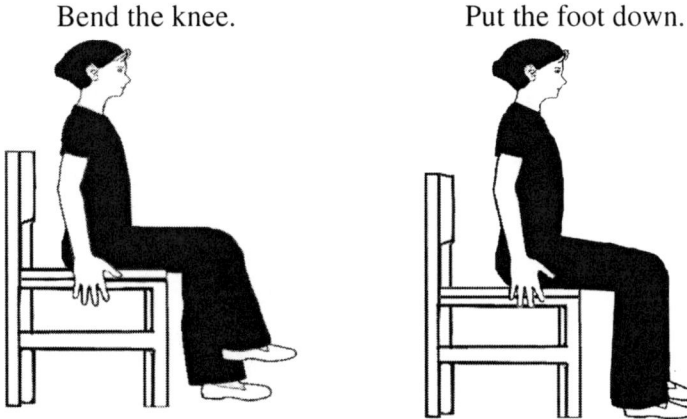

Sit up straight.   Lift the knee.   Straighten the leg.

Bend the knee.   Put the foot down.

Checklist
- Stand or sit up straight. Do as much as you can standing.
- If possible do all repetitions on one leg and then switch to the other leg. If this bothers your hips or back you can alternate legs
- Move through your full range of motion, but do not lock the knee
- Exhale as you lift the leg, inhale as you lower the leg
- Move slowly using a "four thousand count" both to lift the leg and to lower the leg
- Add ankle weights when you feel ready
- Use diaphragmatic breathing through the nose as much as possible
- Do not exercise to the point of strain or discomfort

Side Leg Lift
Muscles worked: Abductors (Hip, outer thigh)
(Tensor fasciae late, gluteus medius, and gluteus minimus)

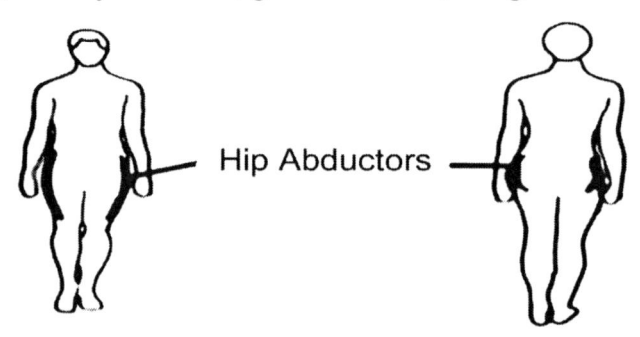

Standing

Before starting, check your posture. Stand up straight, bring the hips under the shoulders, and think about pushing the crown of the head to the ceiling without lifting the chin. Lift the leg straight out to the side as high as you can without tipping the body. Let the heel lead and make the toes face forward or point towards the other leg. Then lower slowly down. *Do not let the leg turn out.* Do eight to twelve repetitions with the right leg, then eight to twelve repetitions with the left leg.

Right Leg

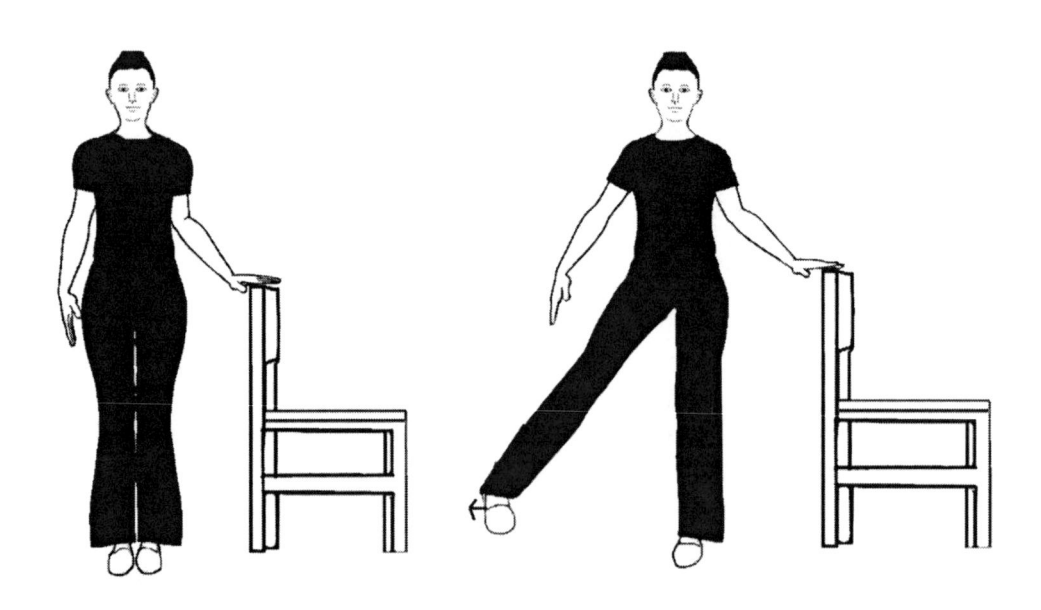

Left Leg

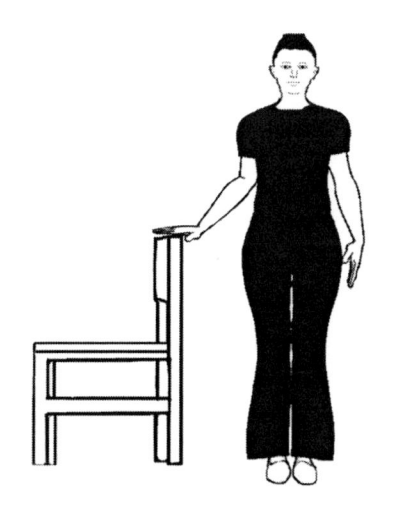

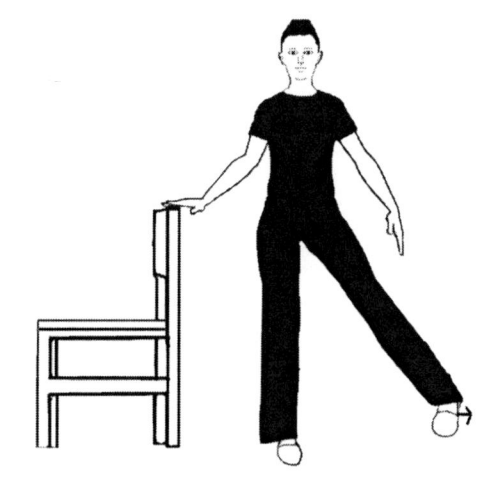

Seated

Sit up straight, away from the back of the chair if possible. If you need to sit back, sit all the way back to avoid slouching. Bring the leg out to the side without swinging the hips. Do eight to twelve repetitions with the right leg and then repeat with the left.

Right Leg   *Left Leg*

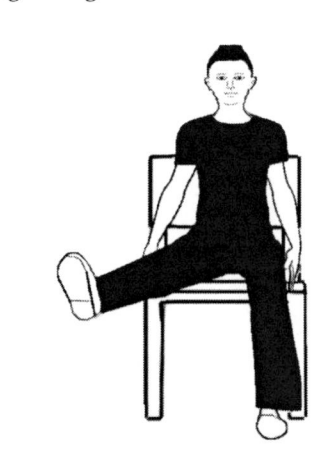

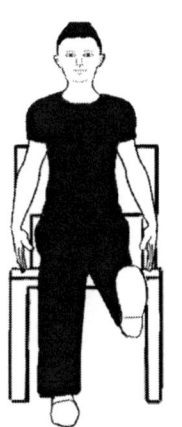

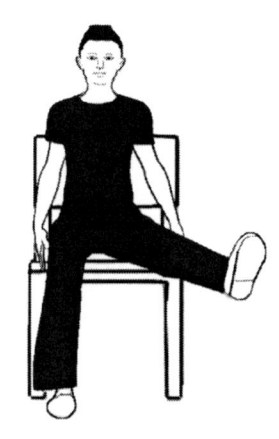

Checklist
- ✓ Stand or sit up straight. Do as much as you can standing
- ✓ If possible do all repetitions on one leg and then switch to the other leg.
- ✓ Move through your full range of motion, but do not swing the hips
- ✓ Exhale as you bring the leg out, inhale as you bring the leg back
- ✓ Move slowly using a "four thousand count" for both movements
- ✓ Add ankle weights when you feel ready
- ✓ Use diaphragmatic breathing through the nose as much as possible
- ✓ Do not exercise to the point of strain or discomfort

Standing Leg Lift Back and Seated Heel Curl
Muscles worked: Gluteal & Hamstring Muscles
(Buttocks, back top of thigh)
(Gluteus maximus, biceps femoris,
semitendinosus, and semimembranosus)

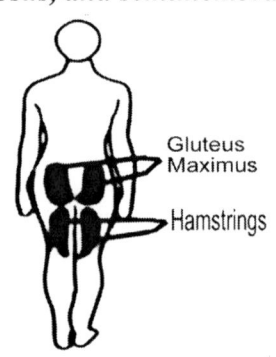

Before starting, check your posture. Stand up straight, hips under the shoulders, and think about pushing the crown of the head to the ceiling without lifting the chin.

Standing

Stand up straight. Tighten the buttocks muscles. Lift the leg directly out to the back. Then lower slowly down. Do not let the leg go out to the side. The toes should point forward. Do not let the shoulders tip forward. Do eight to twelve repetitions with the right leg, then eight to twelve repetitions with the left leg.

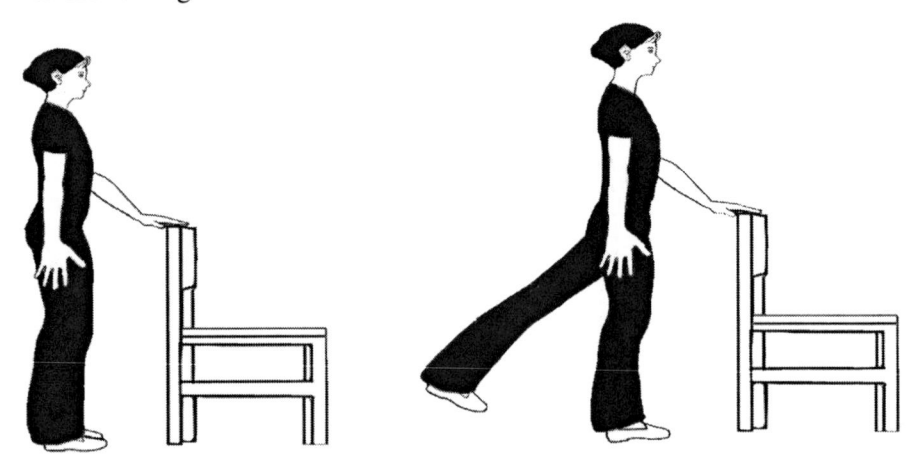

Seated Heel Curl

Sit up straight, away from the back of the chair if possible. If you need to sit back, sit all the way back to avoid slouching. Tighten the muscles in the back top of your thigh and squeeze the heel under the chair, or if your knee is sensitive bring the foot to the outside of the chair. Then return forward slowly. Do eight to twelve repetitions with the right leg, then eight to twelve repetitions with the left leg.

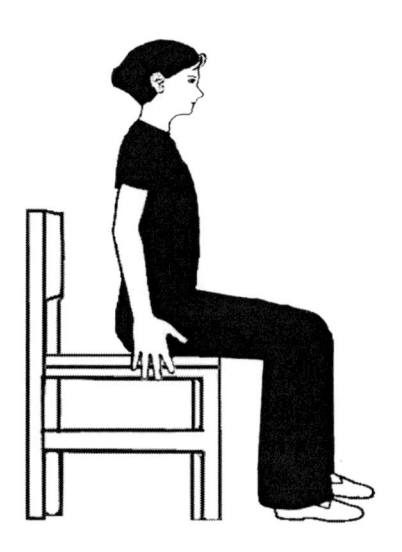

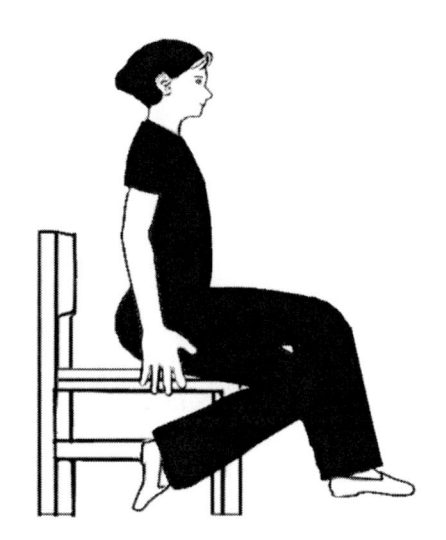

Checklist
- ✓ Stand or sit up straight. Do as much as you can standing
- ✓ Do not let the body tip forward, keep the shoulders over the hips
- ✓ If possible do all repetitions on one leg and then switch to the other leg.
- ✓ If this bothers your hips or back you can alternate legs
- ✓ Move through your full range of motion, but do not swing the hips
- ✓ Exhale as you lift the leg out, inhale as you lower the leg
- ✓ Move slowly using a "four thousand count" for both movements
- ✓ Add ankle weights when you feel ready
- ✓ Use diaphragmatic breathing through the nose as much as possible
- ✓ Do not exercise to the point of strain or discomfort

Stand Leg Crossover
Muscles worked: Adductor Muscles (Inner thigh)
(Adductor longus, adductor brevis, and adductor magnus)

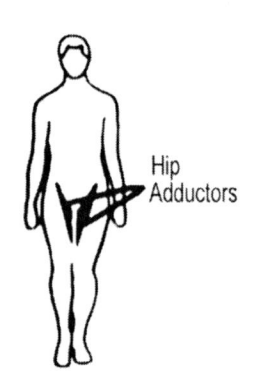

Standing

Before starting, check your posture. Stand up straight, bring the hips under the shoulders, and think about pushing the crown of the head to the ceiling without lifting the chin. Bring your leg across your body. Let the knee bend and drop out to the side and think about lifting your heel up. Then lower slowly down. Do eight to twelve repetitions with the right leg, then eight to twelve repetitions with the left leg.

Right Leg

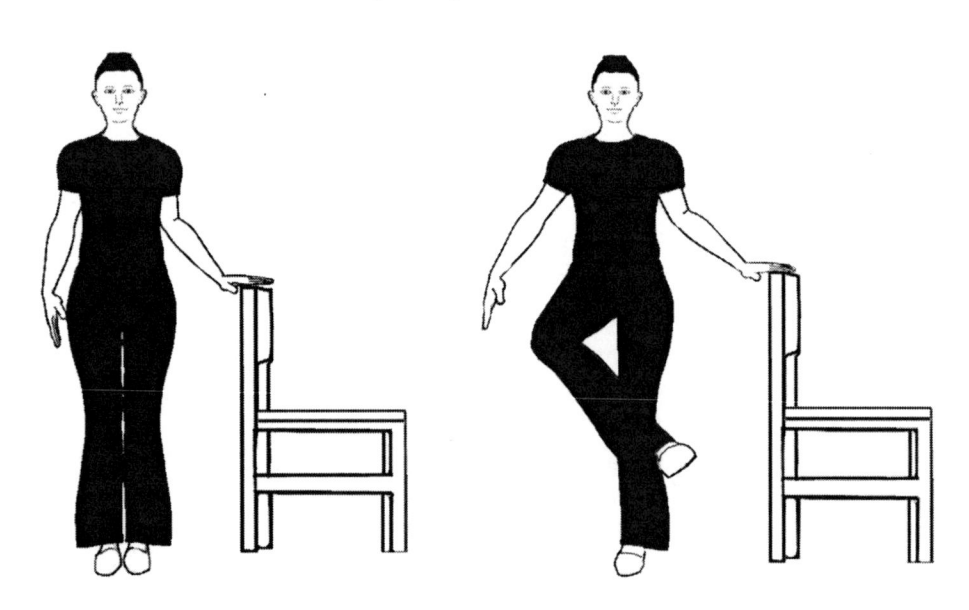

Left Leg

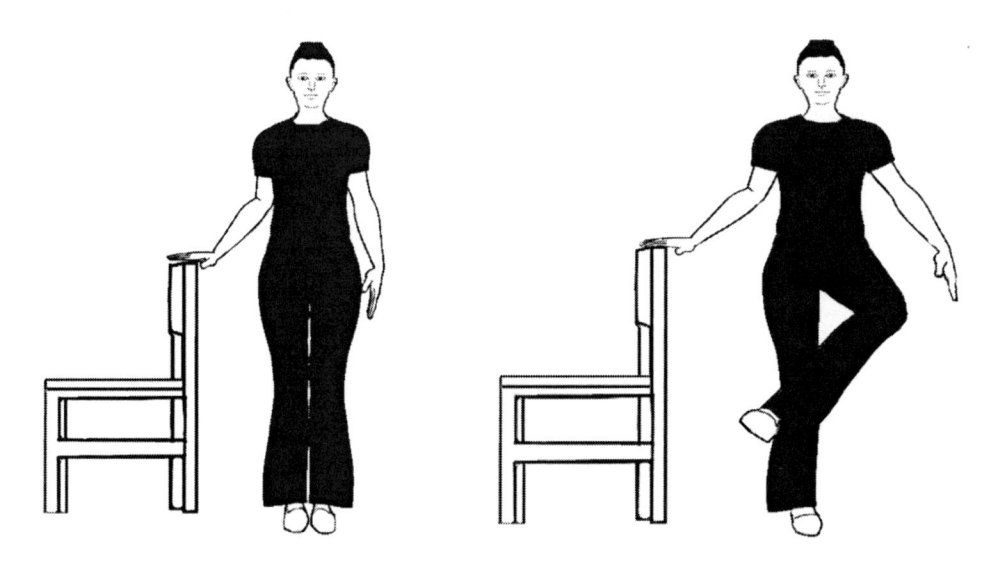

Seated

Sit up straight, away from the back of the chair if possible. If you need to sit back, sit all the way back to avoid slouching. Let the knee bend and drop out to the side and think about lifting your heel up. Then lower slowly down. Do eight to twelve repetitions on the right and then repeat with the left leg.

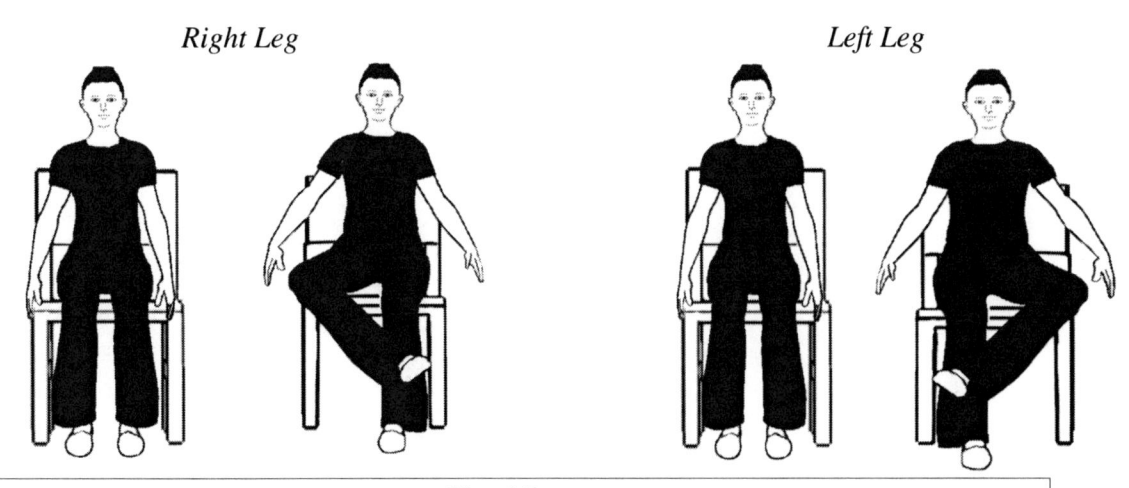

Right Leg   *Left Leg*

Checklist
- ✓ Stand or sit up straight. Do as much as you can standing.
- ✓ If possible do all repetitions on one leg and then switch to the other leg.
- ✓ Exhale as you lift the leg, inhale as you lower the leg
- ✓ Move slowly using a "four thousand count" both to lift the leg and to lower the leg
- ✓ Add ankle weights when you feel ready
- ✓ Do not exercise to the point of strain or discomfort

Heel Raises
Muscles worked: Gastrocnemius and Soleus (Calf)
(Gastrocnemeus when standing and Soleus when seated)

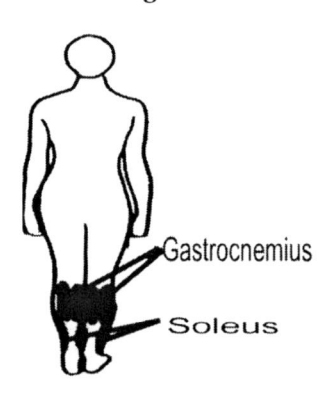

Standing

Before starting, check your posture. Stand up straight, bring the hips under the shoulders, and think about pushing the crown of the head to the ceiling without lifting the chin. Using the chair as little as possible rise up onto the toes. When lowering just barely touch the heels, keeping most of the weight in the toes. Do not drop or bounce down hard. Make sure you do not rock the body back as you land. Keep this movement very small and controlled. Do eight to twelve repetitions.

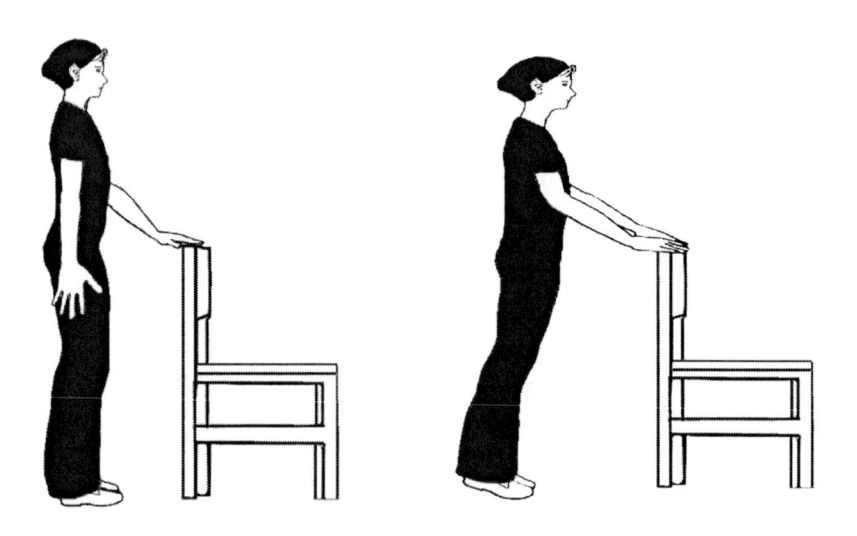

Seated

Sit up straight, away from the back of the chair if possible. If you need to sit back, sit all the way back to avoid slouching. Lift the heels and keep the toes on the floor. When lowering just barely touch the heels, keeping most of the weight in the toes. Do not drop or bounce down hard. Make sure you do not rock the body back as you land. Keep this movement very small and controlled. Do eight to twelve repetitions.

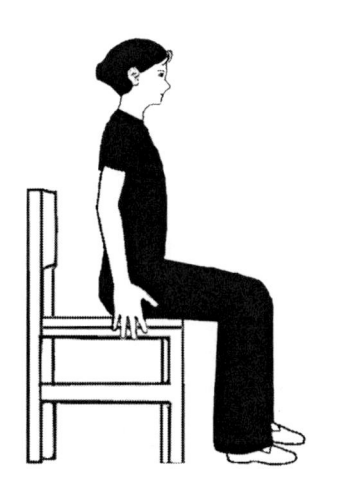

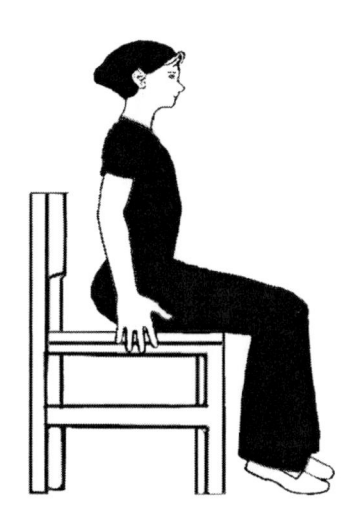

Checklist
- ✓ Stand or sit up straight. Do as much as you can standing.
- ✓ Try to keep the weight in your toes and not back in your heels
- ✓ Move slowly using a "four thousand count" both to lift the heels and to lower the heels
- ✓ Add ankle weights when you feel ready
- ✓ Use diaphragmatic breathing through the nose as much as possible
- ✓ Do not exercise to the point of strain or discomfort

Toe Lifts
Muscles worked: Tibialis Anterior (Shin)

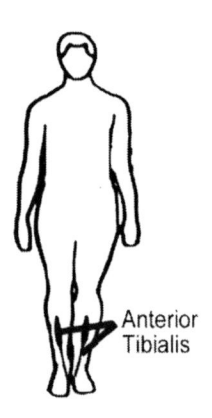

Anterior Tibialis

Standing

Before starting, check your posture. Stand up straight, bring the hips under the shoulders, and think about pushing the crown of the head to the ceiling without lifting the chin. Using the chair as little as possible, bend the knees slightly and lift up just the toes. Then lower slowly down. Make sure you do not rock the hips backwards and keep the heels down. Do eight to twelve repetitions.

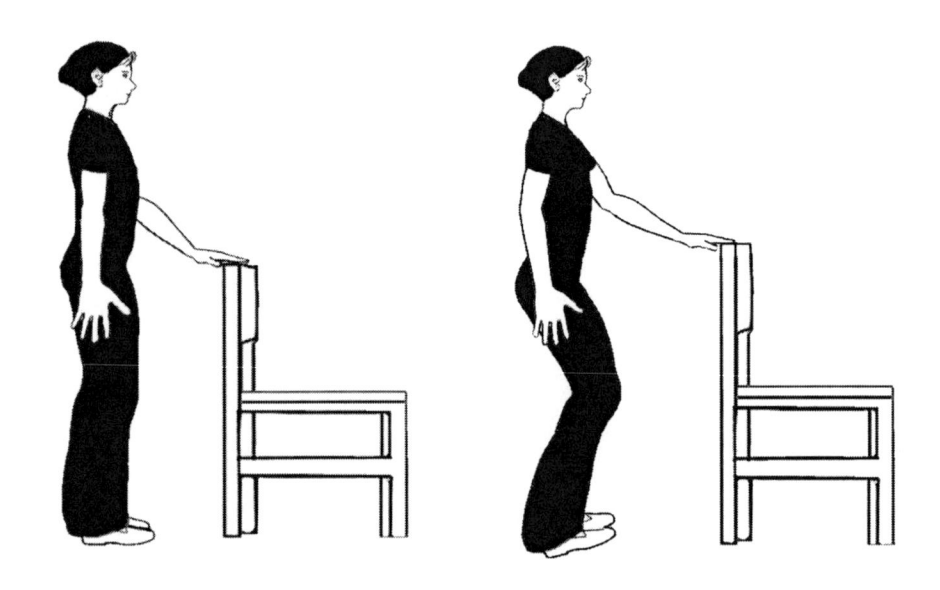

Seated

Sit up straight, away from the back of the chair if possible. If you need to sit back, sit all the way back to avoid slouching. Lift up the toes, keeping the heels down. Then lower slowly down. Make sure you do not rock the hips backwards and keep the heels down. Do eight to twelve repetitions.

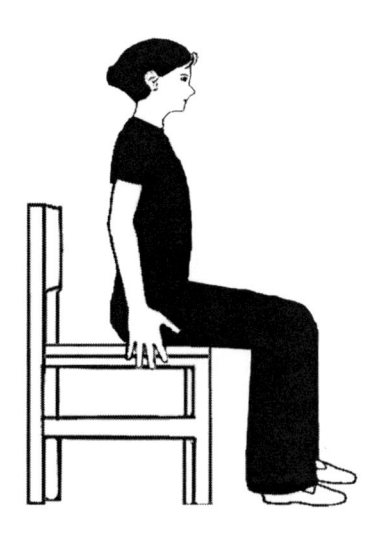

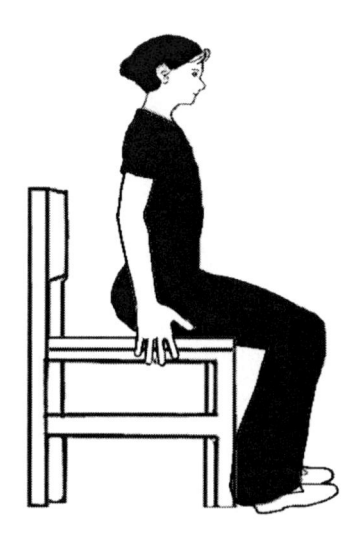

Checklist
- ✓ Stand or sit up straight. Do as much as you can standing
- ✓ Do not rock backwards when lifting the toes
- ✓ Move slowly using a "four thousand count" both to lift and lower the toes
- ✓ Add ankle weights when you feel ready
- ✓ Use diaphragmatic breathing through the nose as much as possible
- ✓ Do not exercise to the point of strain or discomfort

Wall Pushups/Seated Chest Fly
Muscles worked: Pectoralis Major (Chest)

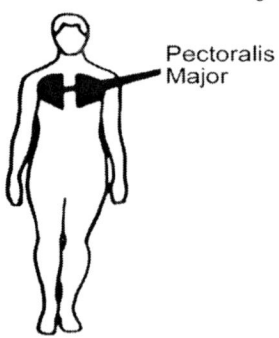

Before starting, check your posture. Stand up straight, bring the hips under the shoulders, and think about pushing the crown of the head to the ceiling without lifting the chin. Stand arms length away from the wall. Place your hands on the wall chest height and shoulder width apart. Bend the elbows and bring your nose and chest as close to the wall as possible, keeping your hips and shoulders in one line. Do not let your hips come forward. Then push back out without locking the elbows. Do eight to twelve repetitions.

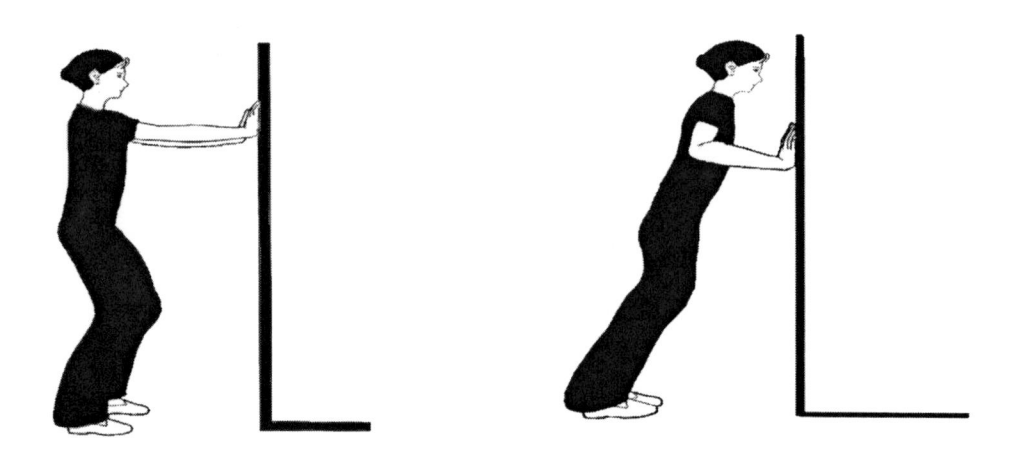

Checklist
- ✓ Keep your body straight, do not drop the hips forward
- ✓ Do not lock the elbows
- ✓ Move slowly using a "four thousand count" for all movements
- ✓ Exhale as you push away from the wall and inhale as you lower in
- ✓ Use diaphragmatic breathing through the nose as much as possible
- ✓ Do not exercise to the point of strain or discomfort

Seated Chest Fly

You can work the same muscles by doing a seated chest fly. Sit at the very front edge of the chair. Then lean back so your upper back touches the chair for support. Do not drop your head back – keep your neck straight and in alignment.

Keeping the elbows slightly bent, open your arms out to the side. Do not let the wrists, hands or weights drop, make sure you control the movement. The bring the weights up in *front of your chest (not your face)* in a circular motion – like you were hugging something. Keep your elbows bent throughout this movement – both when opening the arms and lifting the arms. Exhale as you lift the weights, inhale as you lower them. Do eight to twelve repetitions.

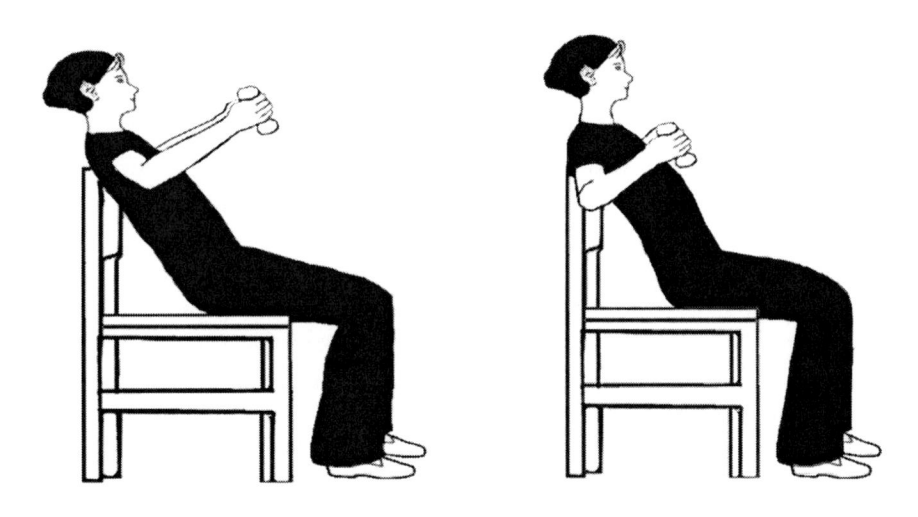

Checklist
- ✓ Lean your upper back only against the back of the chair, keep the abdominal muscles tight to protect your back
- ✓ Do not lock the elbows
- ✓ Keep your arms rounded and the elbows bent throughout, do not drop the hands or wrists back
- ✓ Move slowly using a "4 thousand count" to both lift and lower the weights
- ✓ Exhale as you round forward, inhale as you open the arms
- ✓ Use diaphragmatic breathing through the nose as much as possible
- ✓ Do not exercise to the point of strain or discomfort

Bent Row
Muscles worked: Trapezius, Rhomboids, Latissimus Dorsi
(Upper and mid back)

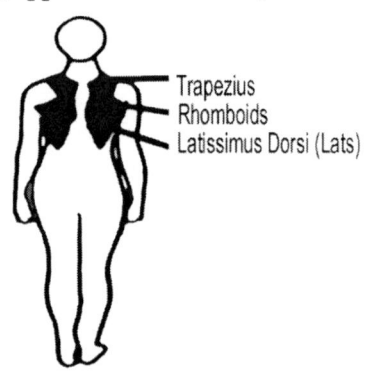

This exercise can be done seated or standing. The seated version may isolate the muscles better but it can place some strain on the back. Try both variations to see which version works best.

Standing

In standing, this exercise is illustrated using just one arm at a time to protect the back. Stand in a lunge and place your left hand on the chair for support. Keep your arm and elbow close to your body and squeeze the shoulder blades together as you lift the right elbow until your hand comes about waist height. Then press the arm down. Keep the abdominal muscles pulled in to protect the back. Do eight to twelve repetitions with the right arm, then eight to twelve repetitions with the left arm.

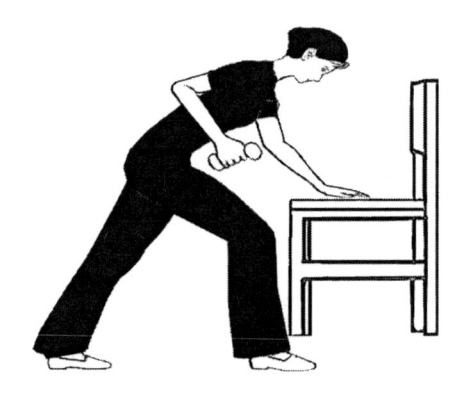

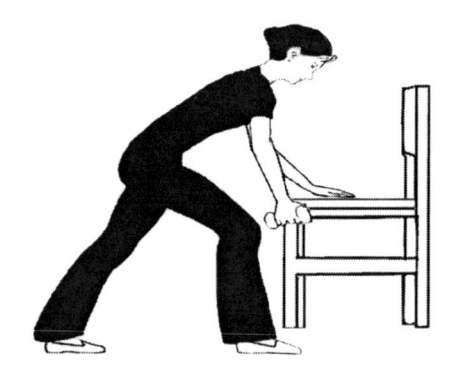

Seated

For the seated version, lean forward from the hips and look down and slightly ahead. Do not lift the head and compress the neck. Tighten the abdominal muscles and squeeze the shoulder blades together as you lift both elbows up until your hands come about waist height. Then press the arm down. Do eight to twelve repetitions.

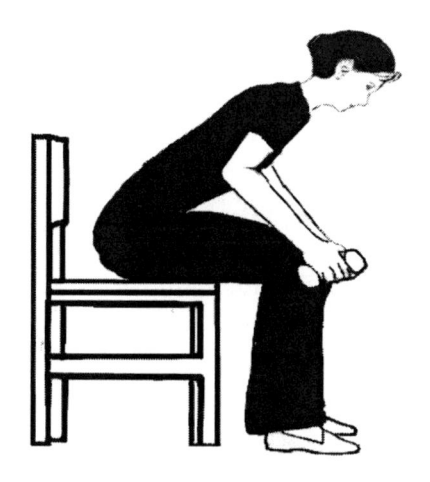

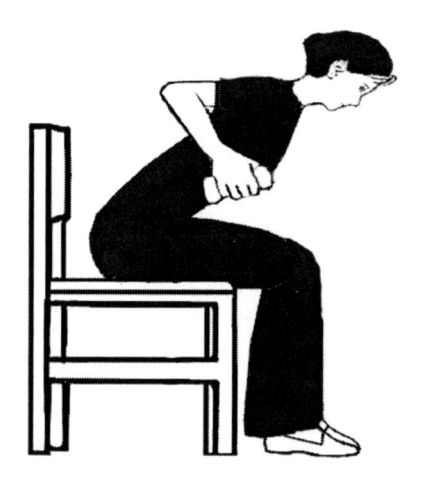

Checklist
- ✓ Keep the abdominal muscles in and the back straight
- ✓ Do not lock the elbows, keep them close to your body and bent when lifting
- ✓ Move slowly using a "4 thousand count" both to lift the weight and to lower the weight
- ✓ Exhale as you lift the weight up, inhale as you lower the weight down
- ✓ Use diaphragmatic breathing through the nose as much as possible
- ✓ Do not exercise to the point of strain or discomfort

Front Lateral Raise
Muscles worked: Deltoid (Shoulders)

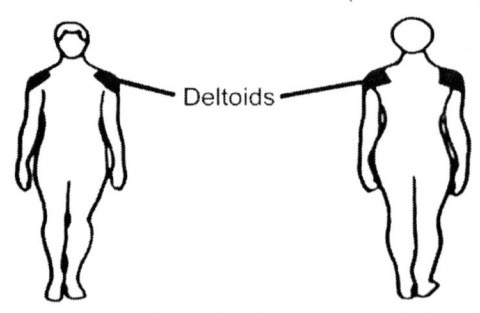

Before starting, check your posture. Sit at the front edge of the chair in order to engage your abdominal muscles. If you need to sit back, sit all the way back in the chair to avoid slouching. Let the arms hang at your sides with the palms facing back. Without rocking the body backwards, exhale and lift the weights up in front of you to *shoulder height only*. Inhale and lower back down. If lifting both arms at the same time bothers your back you can do just one arm at a time. Do eight to twelve repetitions.

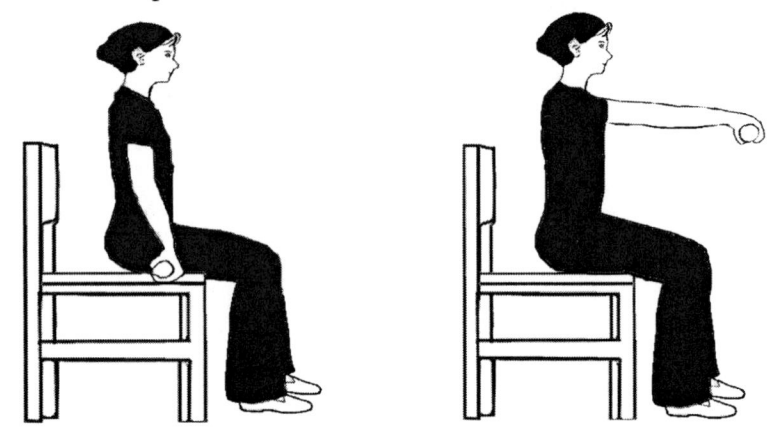

Checklist
- ✓ Sit up straight, away from the back of the chair if possible
- ✓ Exhale as you lift the weight up, inhale as you lower the weight
- ✓ Do not arch your back or rock backwards while lifting the weight and do not lock the elbows
- ✓ Make sure you only lift the weight to shoulder height
- ✓ Move slowly using a "four thousand count" both to lift the weight and to lower the weight
- ✓ Use diaphragmatic breathing through the nose as much as possible
- ✓ Do not exercise to the point of strain or discomfort

Military Press
Muscles worked: Deltoid and Trapezius (Shoulders)

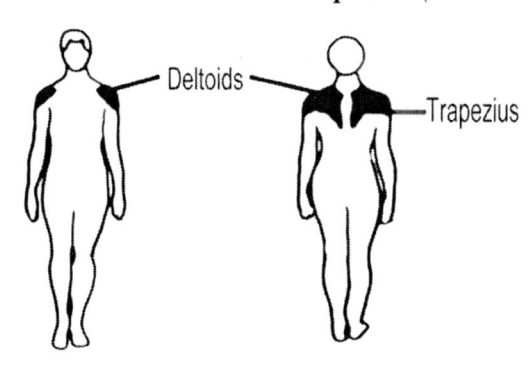

Before starting, check your posture. Sit at the front edge of the chair in order to engage your abdominal muscles. If you need to sit back, sit all the way back to avoid slouching. Bring your hands to shoulder height. Your palms face forward to open the shoulders and prevent forward rounding of the shoulders. Bring the hands back towards the ears as much as possible. Exhale as you lift up and inhale as you lower back to shoulder height. Do not lock your elbows. Do eight to twelve repetitions.

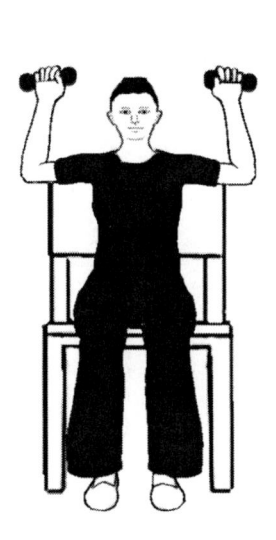

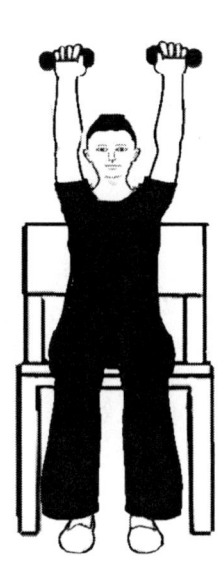

Checklist
- ✓ Sit up straight, away from the back of the chair if possible
- ✓ Exhale as you lift the weight up, inhale as you lower the weight
- ✓ Do not arch your back and do not lock your elbows
- ✓ Move slowly using a "four thousand count" both to lift and lower the weight
- ✓ Use diaphragmatic breathing through the nose as much as possible
- ✓ Do not exercise to the point of strain or discomfort

Deltoid Raise
Muscles worked: Deltoid (Shoulders)

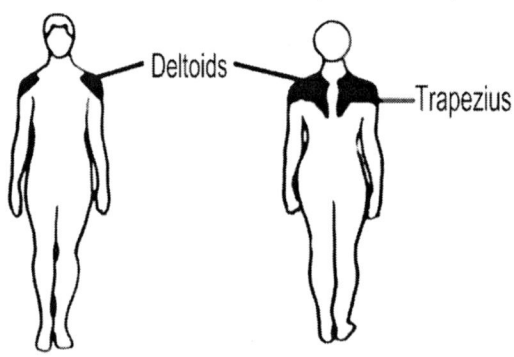

Before starting, check your posture. Sit at the front edge of the chair as much as possible in order to engage your abdominal muscles. If you need to sit back, sit all the way back in the chair to avoid slouching. Bring your hands down by your side. Exhale as you lift straight up to the side, to shoulder height only. Your palms should be facing the floor. Keep your elbows straight but do not lock them. Inhale and lower back down. Do eight to twelve repetitions.

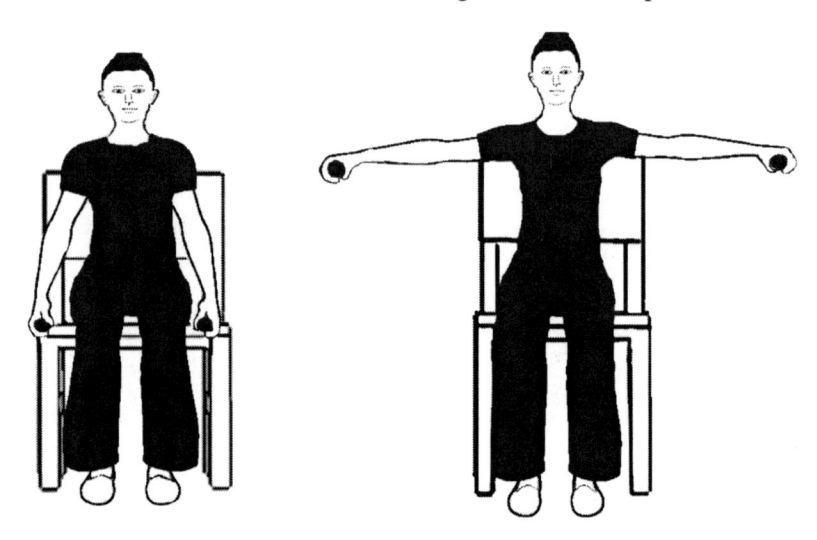

Checklist
- ✓ Sit up straight, away from the back of the chair if possible
- ✓ Exhale as you lift the weight up, inhale as you lower the weight
- ✓ Do not arch your back or rock backwards while lifting and do not lock your elbows
- ✓ Move slowly using a "four thousand count" both to lift and lower the weight
- ✓ Use diaphragmatic breathing through the nose as much as possible
- ✓ Do not exercise to the point of strain or discomfort

Biceps Curl
Muscles worked: Biceps (Front top of arm)

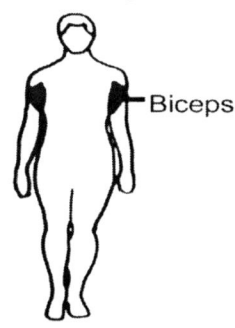

Before starting, check your posture. Sit at the front edge of the chair as much as possible in order to engage your abdominal muscles. If you need to sit back, sit all the way back in the chair to avoid slouching. Bring your hands down by your side. Turn your palms so they face forward. Exhale as you bend your elbows, bringing the weights to your shoulders. Keep your elbows at your side. Do not lift the elbows to bring the weight up. Inhale and lower back down. Do eight to twelve repetitions.

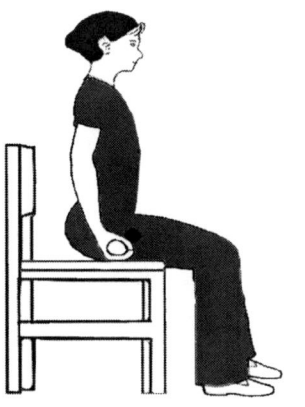

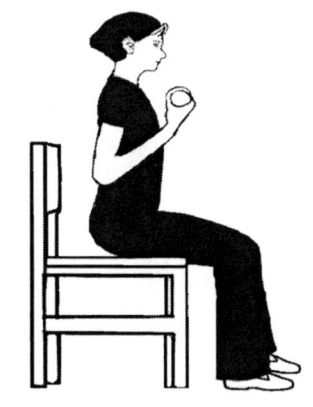

Checklist
- ✓ Sit up straight, away from the back of the chair if possible
- ✓ Exhale as you lift the weight up, inhale as you lower the weight
- ✓ Do not arch your back or rock backwards while lifting and do not lock your elbows
- ✓ Move slowly using a "four thousand count" both to lift and lower the weight
- ✓ Use diaphragmatic breathing through the nose as much as possible
- ✓ Do not exercise to the point of strain or discomfort

Triceps Kickback
Muscles worked: Triceps (Back top of arm)

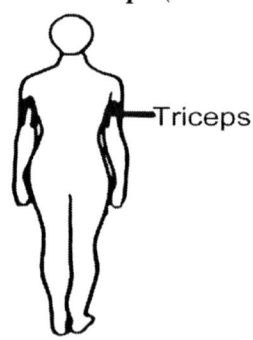

Before starting, check your posture. Sit at the front edge of the chair and tighten your abdominal muscles. Bring your elbows to your sides and lean slightly forward without straining your back. Leaning forward helps to better isolate the muscle. Keep the abdominal muscles tight. Straighten your arms and bring the weights behind you keeping them close to the chair. Then, *just bend at the elbows* to bring the hands back towards your knees. Avoid swinging the whole arm. The movement is just at the elbow joint. If doing both arms at the same time bothers your back you can do just one arm at a time. Do eight to twelve repetitions.

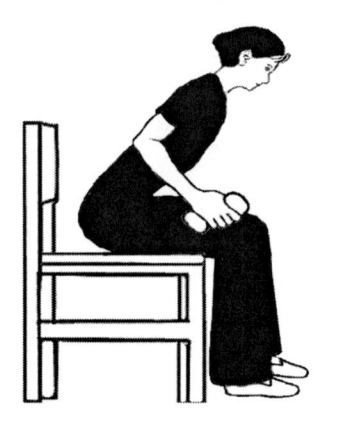

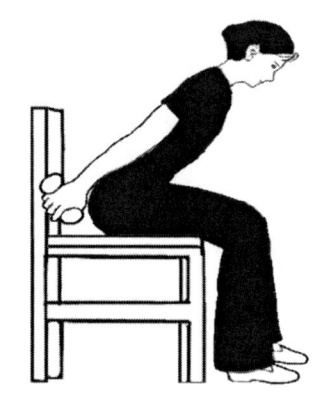

Checklist
- ✓ Exhale as you straighten the elbow, inhale as you bend the elbow
- ✓ Lean forward enough to isolate the muscle, but not too far as to strain the back
- ✓ Do not arch your back or rock backwards while lifting and do not lock the elbow
- ✓ Make sure you just bend and straighten the elbow – do not swing the whole arm
- ✓ Move slowly using a "four thousand count" both to straighten and bend the elbow
- ✓ Use diaphragmatic breathing through the nose as much as possible
- ✓ Do not exercise to the point of strain or discomfort

Wrist Curls
Muscles worked: Flexor Carpi Radialis, Flexor Carpi Ulnaris
(Front of wrists and forearm)

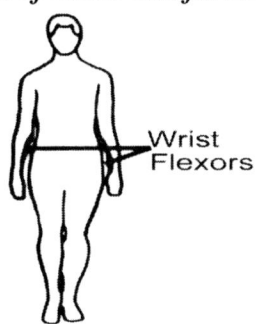

Before starting, check your posture. Sit at the front edge of the chair as much as possible in order to engage your abdominal muscles. Lean forward and place the back of your wrists on your knees. Your hands should be past your knees with the palms facing the ceiling. Exhale as you curl the wrist up. Inhale and curl back down. Keep the movement in the wrist only, do not lift your arms off of your thighs. Do eight to twelve repetitions.

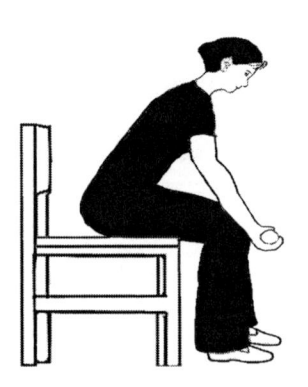

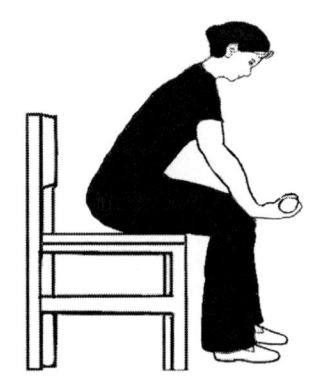

Checklist
- ✓ Lean forward and place your forearm on your knees
- ✓ Exhale as you lift the weight up, inhale as you lower the weight
- ✓ Do not lift your forearm off of your knee as you lift the weight, keep the movement just in the wrist.
- ✓ Move slowly using a "four thousand count" to both lift and lower the weight
- ✓ Use diaphragmatic breathing through the nose as much as possible
- ✓ Do not exercise to the point of strain or discomfort.

Reverse Wrist Curls
Muscles worked: Extensor Carpi Radialis Brevis, Extensor Carpi Ulnaris   (Back of wrists)

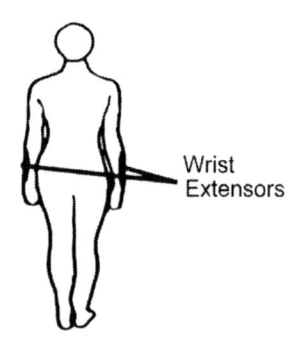

Before starting, check your posture. Sit at the front edge of the chair as much as possible in order to engage your abdominal muscles. Lean forward and place the front of your wrists on your knees. Your hands should be past your knees with the palms facing the floor. Exhale as you curl the wrist up. Inhale and curl back down. Keep the movement in the wrist only, do not lift your arms off of your thighs. Do eight to twelve repetitions.

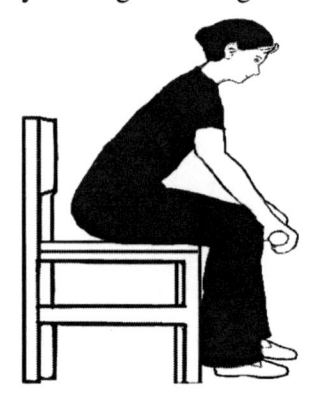

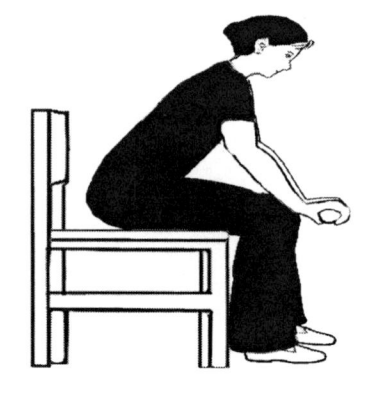

Checklist
- ✓ Lean forward and place your forearm on your knees
- ✓ Exhale as you lift the weight up, inhale as you lower the weight
- ✓ Do not lift your forearm off of your knee as you lift the weight, keep the movement just in the wrist.
- ✓ Move slowly using a "four thousand count" to both lift and lower the weight
- ✓ Use diaphragmatic breathing through the nose as much as possible
- ✓ Do not exercise to the point of strain or discomfort.

Lean Backs
Muscles worked: Rectus Abdominus (Abdominal muscles)

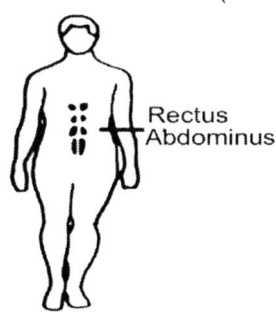

This exercise works the upper abdominal muscles. Sit at the front edge of the chair so you have room to lean back. Cross your arms at your chest. Inhale and sit up straight and let the low back arch slightly. Tuck the chin into the chest and round the low back as you lean back. Go back until you feel a pull in the stomach muscles without touching the chair. Keep the back rounded. If you feel anything in your back instead of in the abdominal muscles, you may be arching your back. Do not drop the head back and keep the shoulders down. Hold back for a five-second count without holding the breath. Inhale and come back up straight. Do eight to twelve repetitions.

Sit up, low back arched   Lean back and hold, chin tucked, back rounded.

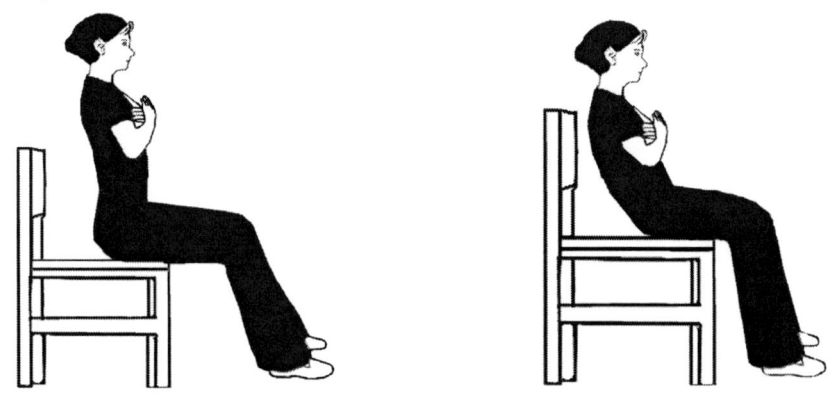

Checklist
- Inhale as you sit up, exhale as you lean back
- You should feel this in your stomach not your back
- Keep the spine slightly rounded and do not drop the head back
- Move slowly using a "four thousand count" both to lean back and to come forward
- Use diaphragmatic breathing through the nose as much as possible
- Do not exercise to the point of strain or discomfort

Bicycles:
Muscles worked: Rectus Abdominus (Abdominal muscles)

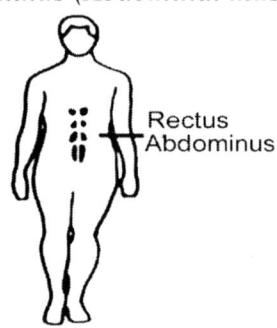

This exercise works the lower abdominal muscles. Before starting, check your posture. Sit at the front edge of the chair so you have room to lean back. Cross your arms at your chest. Inhale as you sit up and let the low back arch slightly. Tuck the chin into the chest, round the back and lean back. Go back until you feel a pull in the abdominal muscles without touching the chair. Keep your back rounded. If you feel anything in your back instead of in the stomach, you may be arching your back. Do not drop the head back and keep the shoulders down. Hold back as you lift either one leg at a time or bicycle the legs for a count of six times. Come back up and repeat. Do not hold your breath. Do five to six repetitions.

Sit up straight. Lean back alternately lifting legs. This version is better for those with sensitive backs.

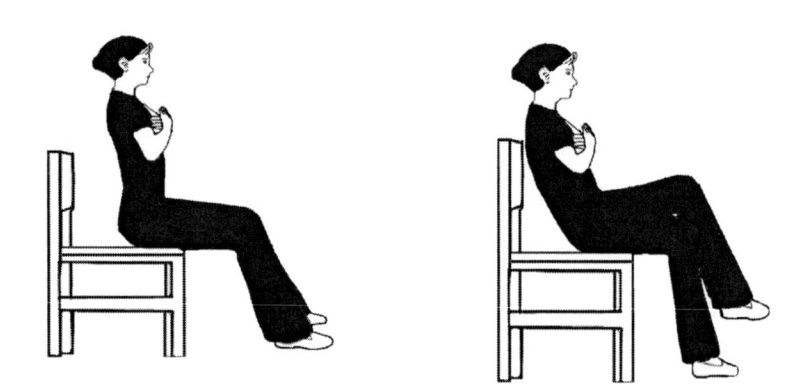

Checklist
- ✓ Keep the spine slightly rounded and the chin tucked in
- ✓ Do not hold your breath. Breathe in and out throughout the exercise
- ✓ Use diaphragmatic breathing through the nose as much as possible
- ✓ Do not exercise to the point of strain or discomfort

Lean back and bicycle both legs about 5 to 6 times. Repeat for 6 to 8 repetitions. This is a more challenging variation.

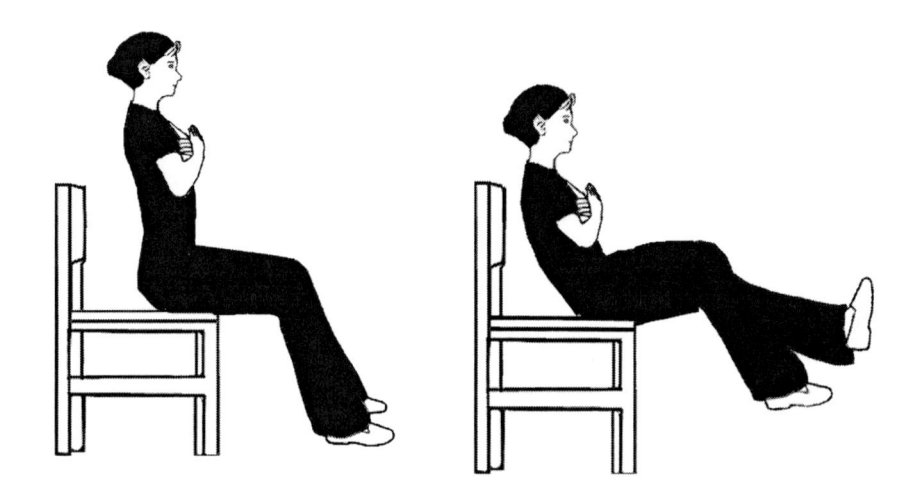

Checklist
- ✓ Keep the spine slightly rounded
- ✓ Do not drop the head back, keep the chin tucked
- ✓ If you feel this exercise in your back instead of your abdominals you are probably arching your back. Focus on pulling the stomach muscles in and keeping the back rounded
- ✓ Do not hold your breath. Breathe in and out throughout the exercise
- ✓ Use diaphragmatic breathing through the nose as much as possible
- ✓ Do not exercise to the point of strain or discomfort

Side Bends
Muscles worked: Obliques (Waist)

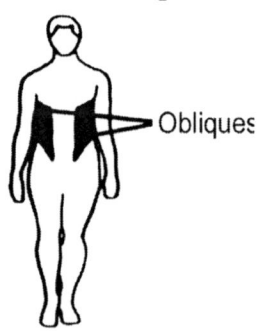

Before starting, check your posture. Sit at the front edge of the chair as much as possible in order to engage your abdominal muscles. Inhale as you sit up straight. Exhale and bend to the right as far as you can. *Do not lean forward*, keep the shoulders over the hips. The elbows stay straight. As you come back up, let the waist muscles lift you up, and do not lift the weight with the arm. Keep the shoulders down and relaxed. Do eight to twelve repetitions on the right, then eight to twelve repetitions on the left.

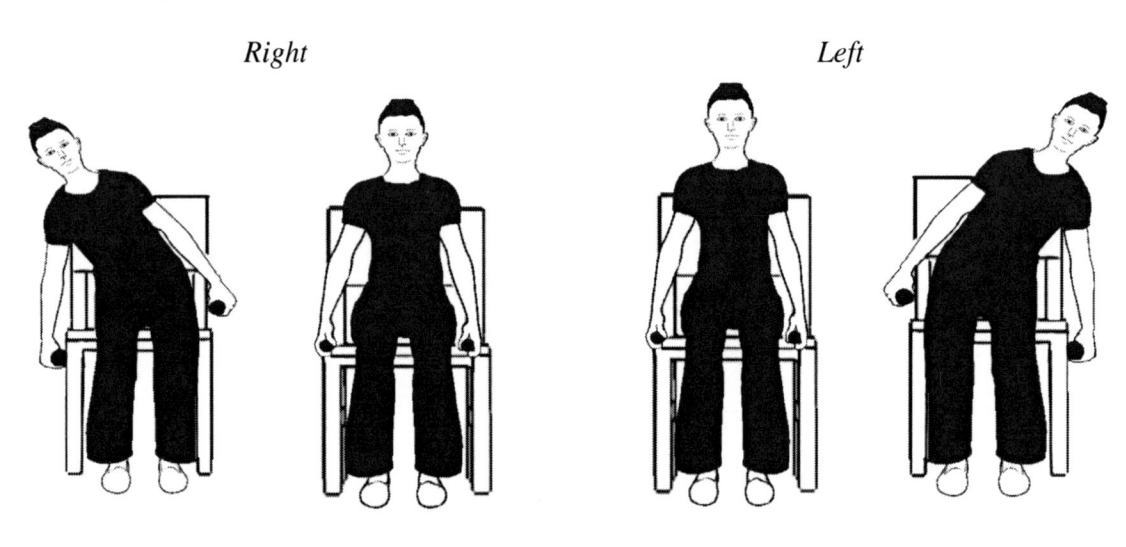

Right *Left*

Checklist
- ✓ Sit up straight, away from the back of the chair if possible
- ✓ Inhale as you sit up, exhale as you bend
- ✓ Keep the shoulders over the hips – do not bend forward, keep the elbows straight
- ✓ Move slowly using a "4 thousand count" both to bend to the side and to sit up straight
- ✓ Use diaphragmatic breathing through the nose as much as possible
- ✓ Do not exercise to the point of strain or discomfort

Summary

There are many other exercises that work the same muscle groups, and many variations on the above exercises. There are also strengthening exercises that can be done using theraband, tubing, and physioballs, and your own body weight. The exercises listed in this chapter demonstrate a safe and complete workout and provide a good starting point. However, following the same exercise routine for long periods will eventually cause your body to adapt to the exercises, and you will discontinue getting good results. It is important to vary your exercise routine from time to time, trying different exercises and different forms of resistance.

After you become familiar with the various muscles you are trying to isolate and you become comfortable using resistance, try looking into other books, videos or classes to help vary your routine. When following any exercise program, remember to use good body mechanics and good form in order to protect your back and joints from injury.

Remember, resistance exercises should always be done slowly and with control.

The next chapter will cover some general yoga postures and tai chi exercises that will help to increase your flexibility, improve your balance and reduce your risk for falls. Yoga and Tai Chi are great ways to increase your awareness of how you are using your body so you can make safer choices and avoid accidents.

> "We have lived in our home for so long, raised our kids here and have so many memories. As my legs became weaker from the PD, getting up and down the stairs started to become too difficult and I thought we were going to have to move. Within just a few months of starting this class I could feel my legs getting stronger and I am now able to go right up the stairs with no problem. We can now remain in the home we love."
> - D.G. Massachusetts.

Chapter 5

Yoga and Tai Chi for Flexibility and Balance

Have patience with all things, but chiefly have patience with yourself.
Do not lose courage in considering your own imperfections but instantly
set about remedying them – every day begin the task anew.
Saint Francis de Sales

Balance problems are common in those with Parkinson's disease and they can increase the risk of a fall. Current statistics by the National Institute for Aging suggest that each year, about one-third of individuals sixty-five years of age or older will fall. These falls often fracture a bone, dislocate a joint, or cause some other serious injury. Sadly many never fully recover, and as a result they permanently lose their ability to function independently. This often leads to placement in a nursing home. In addition, each year approximately 9,500 fall-related deaths occur in older Americans. Given the above, falls and the injuries that result are one of the most substantial health threats facing older Americans.

This chapter will introduce some simple yoga postures and Tai chi movements that when practiced regularly will help to improve your balance and reduce your risk of a fall. As you work to hold the postures your muscles will become stronger. As you continue to stretch and improve your flexibility, everyday tasks will become less challenging which can also decrease your risk for a fall. Another benefit of yoga is that it encourages you to be mindful of how you are using your body. As you become more aware of where your center of gravity is, you will become better at knowing when you are starting to lose your balance and know how to correct it.

Causes of Falls

Falls often occur due to medications such as sedatives, muscle relaxants, and blood pressure drugs, which can cause dizziness, lightheadedness, or loss of balance. When two or more medications are used in combination, these side effects may be exaggerated. Other causes include diminished vision, hearing, muscle strength, coordination, and reflexes. Certain diseases can also affect balance. Falls often occur at home and are common when getting in and out of a chair or shower, stepping backwards and reaching out too far to grab onto something. Many times people who have fallen fear falling again so they restrict their activities. However, as activities are restricted the body loses even more strength and mobility. This leads to more falls, beginning a downward spiral. Instead of becoming less active, those with balance concerns should be encouraged to do exercises that improve balance and strength. This will help in maintaining function, thereby reducing the risk of falling.

Good balance is important to help you get around, remain independent, and carry out daily activities. Having good balance means being able to control and maintain your body's position whether you are moving or remaining still. An intact sense of balance helps you walk without staggering, rise from a chair without falling, and climb stairs more easily.

How Your Body Maintains Balance

The body maintains balance by coordinating information received from three systems – vestibular (hearing), visual, and proprioceptive. The vestibular system works with the visual system to keep objects in focus when the head is moving. The proprioceptive system is comprised of joint and muscle receptors throughout the body that send signals to the brain to aid in maintaining balance. The brain receives, interprets, and processes the information from all of these systems in order to control balance.

The Role of the Vestibular or Auditory System

This system helps maintain balance by sensing the movement and position of the head, and acceleration and deceleration of the body. This occurs through the semicircular canals which are three tiny, fluid-filled tubes in your inner ear. Movement of fluid in the semicircular canals signals the brain about the direction, speed, and rotation of the head, such as when nodding up and down or looking from right to left. When the head moves, the liquid inside the semicircular canals also moves. This in turn puts pressure on the tiny hairs that line each canal. These hairs translate the movement of the liquid into nerve messages that are sent to your brain. Your brain then can tell your body how to stay balanced.

The Role of the Visual System

This system sends visual signals to the brain about the body's position in relation to its surroundings. These signals are processed by the brain, and compared to information from the vestibular and the proprioceptive systems. The visual system provides the brain with visual cues which are utilized as reference points in orienting the body in space.

The Role of the Proprioceptive System

This system provides an information link between your brain and the more than 650 muscles that move your body. This system relies on feedback from skin pressure and muscle and joint sensory receptors to tell the brain what part of the body is touching the ground and what parts of the body are moving. This system is made up of receptor cells found within each muscle fiber and nerves that travel from the muscles through the spinal cord to the brain. This system utilizes specific communication patterns within the brain that interprets these signals, allowing your body to meet the ever-changing demands of movement and balance. When this system is functioning efficiently an individual's body position is automatically adjusted in different situations. The proprioceptive system is responsible for providing the body with the necessary signals to allow us to plan and execute different motor tasks such as sitting properly in a chair and stepping off a curb smoothly. It also allows the body to coordinate fine motor movements such as writing with a pencil, using a spoon to drink soup, and buttoning one's shirt. In order for this system to work properly, it must rely on obtaining accurate information from the sensory systems and then organizing and interpreting this information efficiently and effectively.

Acting together, these three systems constantly gather and interpret sensory information from all over the body. This allows the body to act on that information in an appropriate and helpful way. The information from these systems travels to the central balance mechanism in your brain. In turn, the brain sends out signals allowing you to control your body movements, maintain your balance, and give you a sense of stability.

With age there are natural changes that occur that can affect balance. The fluid inside the ears can begin to dry out and the hairs can become less sensitive. Vision also often diminishes with age and the sensory receptors in the body lose some of their sensitivity. All of the above reduces the information that reaches the brain which can result in a diminished ability to maintain balance. Unfortunately these types of changes can not be avoided. However, even with these changes falls are not considered a normal part of aging and there are steps that can be taken to improve balance at any age. This includes being mindful about body mechanics as discussed in chapter one and keeping the body strong and flexible. A strong and flexible body can better adapt to movement and make the necessary corrections to keep the body balanced.

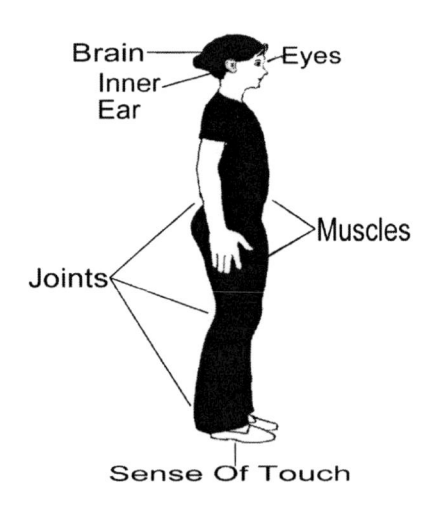

Parkinson's Disease and Your Balance

For many with Parkinson's disease balance is a concern. As mentioned earlier in this chapter the medications you take can affect your body's ability to balance as they can make you tired or less alert. Parkinson's disease itself can also hinder your ability to make adjustments to your body if you start to lose your balance. Having PD can cause freezing or have trouble initiating movement. This means that you may know that you are falling but you may be unable to initiate a movement (such as putting your arm out or taking a step) to stop your fall. In addition the stiffness in the trunk area of the body common in those with PD, may cause you to walk and stand with a bent posture that brings the body out of alignment. If you stand or walk with the head forward and upper back rounded your body weight is uneven and more to the front. When you start to fall forward it will be hard to get yourself back upright and prevent a fall.

Unfortunately, you can not avoid the side effects of your medication but you should be aware of how your meds are affecting you and avoid challenging movements when you are tired or less alert. In addition, there are other steps you can take to help prevent falls. To review from Chapter one, when walking remember to take long strides and let your heel strike first. Avoid scuffing the feet and catching the toes, both of which can trigger a fall. Also make a conscious effort to swing your opposite arm to leg instead of holding the arms stiff. This will help to provide momentum and maintain balance. In all of your daily activities keep reminding yourself to stand up straight and keep the shoulders lined up directly over the hips to maintain your center of gravity. Lastly, regular exercise can help to keep you strong and limber and lessen the risk for a fall.

How Yoga and Tai Chi Can Help Improve Your Balance

Age-related falls are caused in part by a reduced sense of balance and a loss of ability to judge body placement. Aging causes many changes in the body that can increase the chances of a fall. One change is a loss of hearing and less sensitivity in the auditory system. Changes in vision will lessen the information that the brain receives in order to keep the body straight. A loss of sensitivity in the proprioceptors can also occur. As the sensitivity of these systems diminishes the brain is left with less of the sensory information it needs to maintain balance. Slower reflexes, decreased muscle strength, loss of eyesight and depth perception all contribute to a diminished sense of equilibrium. Changes in balance can also be the result of a sedentary lifestyle. Failure to exercise regularly results in poor muscle tone, decreased strength, and loss of bone mass and flexibility. All of these changes not only increase the likelihood of a fall but can also have an impact on the severity of any injury that might occur as a result of a fall.

Maintaining balance requires stability of the core muscles and the joints, particularly the hip, knee, and ankle. With age these areas often decline in muscle strength and size. Performing balance exercises challenges the nervous and muscular systems. As with any system in the body, when it is challenged it can improve. Regular balance training can improve one's strength, coordination, and muscle-reaction times.

The aerobic exercises in chapter three help to improve balance, as they challenge the body to move in a variety of directions at a quick pace, which can help to improve your reflexes. The strength training exercises in chapter four improve muscular strength which will provide stability. The yoga and tai chi movements in this chapter introduce static postures which will improve the body's ability to maintain balance while in various positions. While you may initially find these exercises challenging, with constant practice you will find your balance improving, thereby reducing your risk of a fall.

Flexibility and Range of Motion

Flexibility refers to the ability to move the joints and muscles through their full range of motion. Daily stretching can help to combat the muscle rigidity which accompanies Parkinson's disease. As you become more flexible and gain greater range of motion, you will find it easier to perform everyday activities such as reaching items on high shelves, looking behind you to back up the car, or tying your shoes. The less you have to struggle to perform these activities, the less likely you are to fall and be injured. A regular stretching routine will lead to increased range of motion in the joints, better posture, protection against muscle injuries such as strains or sprains, improved circulation, and a reduction in muscle tension.

Tips for Safe Stretching

- Stretch only to the point where you feel a gentle pull.
- Do not stretch to the point of pain.
- *Do not bounce while you stretch.* Bouncing can cause small tears in the muscle fibers creating less flexibility.
- Do not hold your breath while you stretch. Breathe evenly in-and-out during each stretch.
- Hold each stretch approximately twenty to thirty seconds

One benefit of stretching is that it increases the length of both your muscles and tendons, leading to an increase in range of movement. A flexible joint has the ability to move through a greater range of motion while requiring less energy to do so. Daily stretching improves muscular balance and posture. Stretching also increases joint synovial fluid, which is a lubricating fluid that promotes the transport of more nutrients to the joints' articular cartilage. This allows a greater range of motion and can reduce joint degeneration. Improved muscle coordination is another benefit of regular stretching.

The Benefits of a Yoga Practice

The practice of yoga is often misunderstood by many. The thought of yoga often conjures up thoughts of having to sit cross legged on the floor for long periods, standing on one's head, chanting, being connected with a particular religion or spiritual belief, or wrapping oneself into a posture which seems impossible for the average human to do. Yoga is not about achieving advanced postures, sitting still for long periods, or being connected to a specific religious practice. The word yoga, taken from the Sanskrit word *"Yuj,"* simply means union; union of mind, body and spirit or soul, nothing more. The goal of yoga is to become more connected with your body and mind through the use of movement, breathwork, and meditation or directed concentration.

The practice of yoga can help improve balance, increase flexibility, reduce stress, lower blood pressure, and aids in lessening common aches and pains. Yoga can be especially beneficial for those with injuries or chronic illness. Since yoga is about union of mind, body, and spirit, the main goal for the yoga student is to find the expression of the posture that best suits his or her individual and unique needs. It is about both a willingness to go inside to discover the movements that are best, and a willingness to honor those discoveries. Many traditional yoga postures can be adapted to accommodate all abilities, levels and ages. There are chair yoga classes in which every movement is performed sitting in a chair, and there are also programs for those who are bedridden. Yoga does not require one to follow any specific belief system to participate. The philosophies of yoga are universal and can be incorporated within any belief system. The warm up exercises introduced in chapter two are common movements used in yoga.

Yoga can be a wonderful form of exercise, due to its slow and gentle nature. Many of the postures help improve balance and reduce the risk of falls. As the student of yoga gently and with respect for the body begins to increase flexibility, aches and pains in the back, knees, and hips may lessen as the muscles are stretched and the pressure exerted on the joints is reduced.

Also, as flexibility increases, many of the activities of daily life become easier. When the muscles of the neck loosen it becomes easier to turn the head when trying to back up the car. When the muscles of the legs and back become more limber it becomes easier to reach or pick up items at varying heights. With an increased range of motion in the shoulder muscles, grooming and dressing tasks can become easier. As mentioned earlier the easier your everyday tasks become the less likely you are to fall.

Some of the benefits of a yoga practice include:
- Increased feelings of relaxation. Gentle stretching, breathing, meditation and guided relaxation releases body tension and calms the nervous system and emotions.
- Improved balance. Better focus, attention, and concentration are promoted through a yoga practice of mindful movement and enhanced body awareness. As you gain more body awareness you will be better able to judge when you are out of balance and can make corrections to prevent a fall. Muscles become more toned as they work to hold the yoga postures.
- Improved flexibility. Yoga gently stretches the muscles in the body increasing the flexibility and length of the muscles, tendons and ligaments.
- Improved energy levels. The slow, gentle movements combined with deep breathing help to energize the body.
- Lung capacity can improve. Yoga emphasizes deep diaphragmatic breathing that can help to strengthen the lungs and improve respiratory health.

Yoga Breathing

An important component of yoga is the combination of deep breathing and movement. By paying attention to your breath as you hold the postures will help you learn to release tension in the body and stretch to the appropriate level. This breathing is the same breath introduced in Chapter two and you should be familiar with this technique as it is the same breathing you have been using with all of the exercises in this book. See pages 48-50 to review this breathing technique if needed.

The Poses

Before beginning this sequence of yoga postures it is important to warm up the body. Performing the yoga-based warm-up exercises in chapter two would be a good predecessor to the following movements. For all of the following postures *remember*, that yoga is about honoring the body's needs. With each posture, experiment to find a level of intensity where you are challenging yourself but not struggling. If the breathing becomes restricted or the only thought you have is how soon you can release the posture, you are pushing yourself too hard. If you find the above happening, lessen the stretch or come out of the posture sooner.

As with many of the movements in this book, the yoga postures will be shown standing, standing while holding on, and seated. Try to do as many postures as you can standing without holding on to begin to help improve your balance.

Mountain Pose

Check your posture before you begin. Shoulders should be back and down and over the hips. Knees should remain slightly bent. Tuck in the chin and think about pushing the crown of the head up to the ceiling without lifting your chin. The abdominal muscles are lightly pulled in, but not so much that it restricts your breathing.

Stand up straight and lift your arms up overhead with the palms facing each other. Bring the arms back so the elbows are in line with the ears if possible. Drop the shoulders and line the shoulders up over the hips. Keep the knees slightly bent and the natural curve in the low back. Toes point straight forward. Place equal weight on both feet. Check that there is equal weight on the outside and inside of the foot, and on all of the toes so you are not rolling your ankles in or out. Check that there is equal weight on the ball and heel of the foot so you are not leaning forward or back. Hold for five to ten deep belly breaths or for as long as is comfortable.

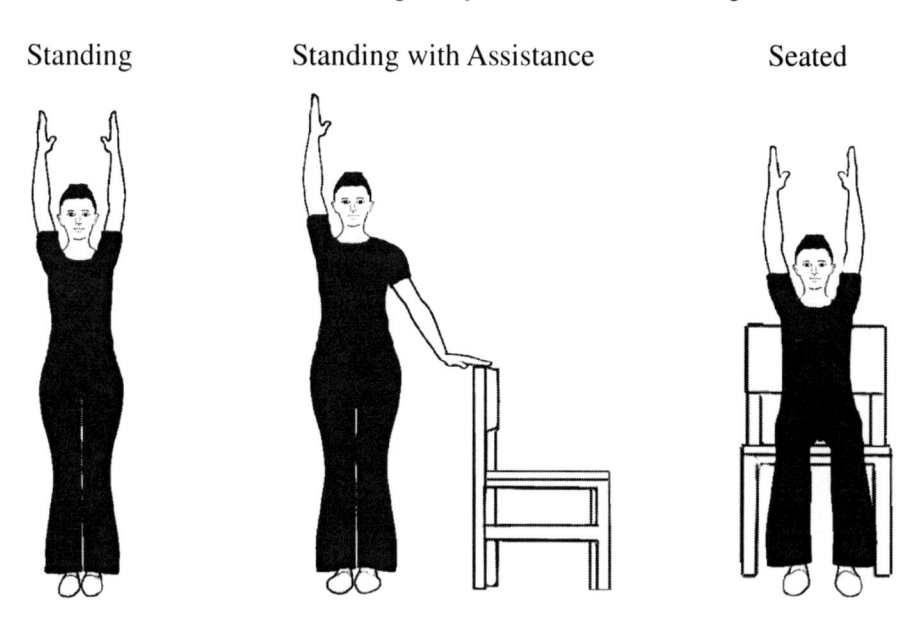

Standing   Standing with Assistance   Seated

Checklist
- Stand or sit up straight. Do as much as you can standing
- Keep the spine straight and the shoulders over the hips
- Keep the shoulders down away from the ears
- Keep the natural curve in the low back
- Hold for five to ten deep belly breaths, or to comfort
- Use diaphragmatic breathing through the nose as much as possible
- Do not exercise to the point of strain or discomfort
- Remember the goal of yoga is to find that point where you are challenging yourself but not struggling

Standing Sway Exercises: Forward and Back and Side to Side

 The purpose of the next two exercises is to improve your reflexes and to help you become aware of when you are putting yourself at risk for a fall. For those with balance concerns it can be tempting to reach too far out in front of you to grab onto a chair or railing for support. However, this brings the head and shoulders ahead of the hips which brings you out of balance. It is much safer to move slowly towards the chair or railing, and not overextend your reach. These exercises will help you discover just how far you can lean forward and back and how far you can reach out to the side without falling. Use these exercises as a way to test your balance. As you discover how far you can lean without falling, remember this limit during daily activities, and never reach out further then you can safely keep your balance. This exercise is only shown standing, as a seated version will not test your balance as well.

 Check your posture before you begin. Shoulders should be back and down and over the hips. Knees are slightly bent. Tuck in the chin and push the crown of the head up to the ceiling without lifting your chin. Lightly contract the abdominal muscles, but not so much that it restricts your breathing.

 Using a chair for safety, stand with your feet shoulder-width apart and your hands resting *lightly* on the chair. Gently lean forward until you feel your toes grab the floor. Then lean backward so that your weight shifts to your heels, and the toes lift slightly. Keep the body stiff. Be sure that your shoulders and hips move together. Do not bend at your hips or waist. Test how far you can sway forward and backward without taking a step, but do not make yourself unsafe. Sway a few times forward and back.

Start Center   Sway Forward   Sway Back

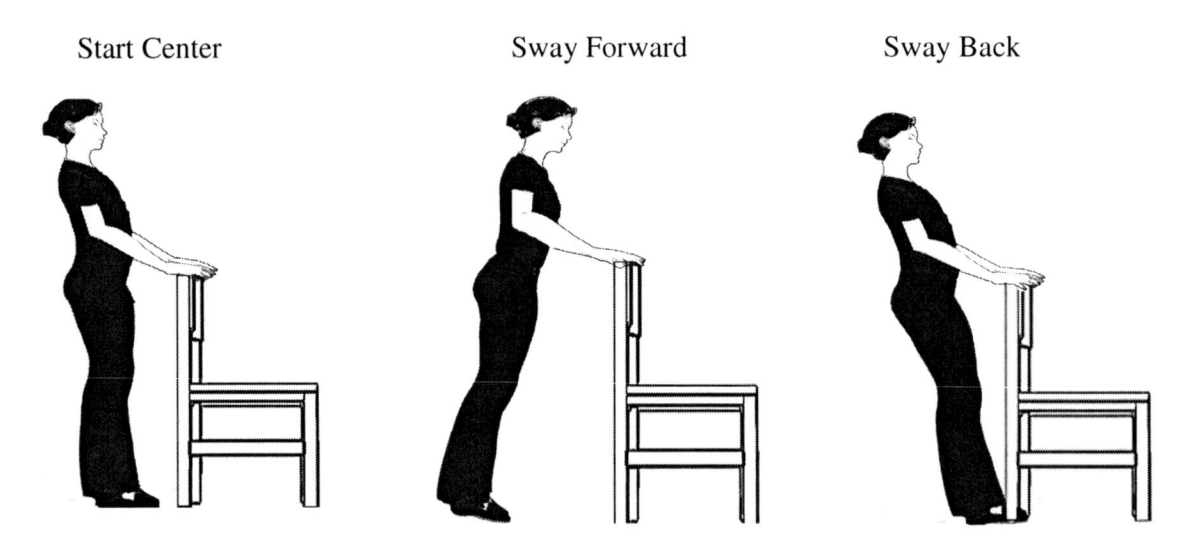

Standing Sway Exercise: Side to Side

Stand with your feet shoulder-width apart and your arms at your side. Gently lean to the right so that all of your weight shifts from your left foot to your right foot. If possible you can lift the left foot slightly. Be sure that your shoulders and hips move together. Do not bend at your hips or waist. Then lean to the left. Slowly increase how far you can sway left and right without taking a step, but do not make yourself unsafe. Sway a few times side to side.

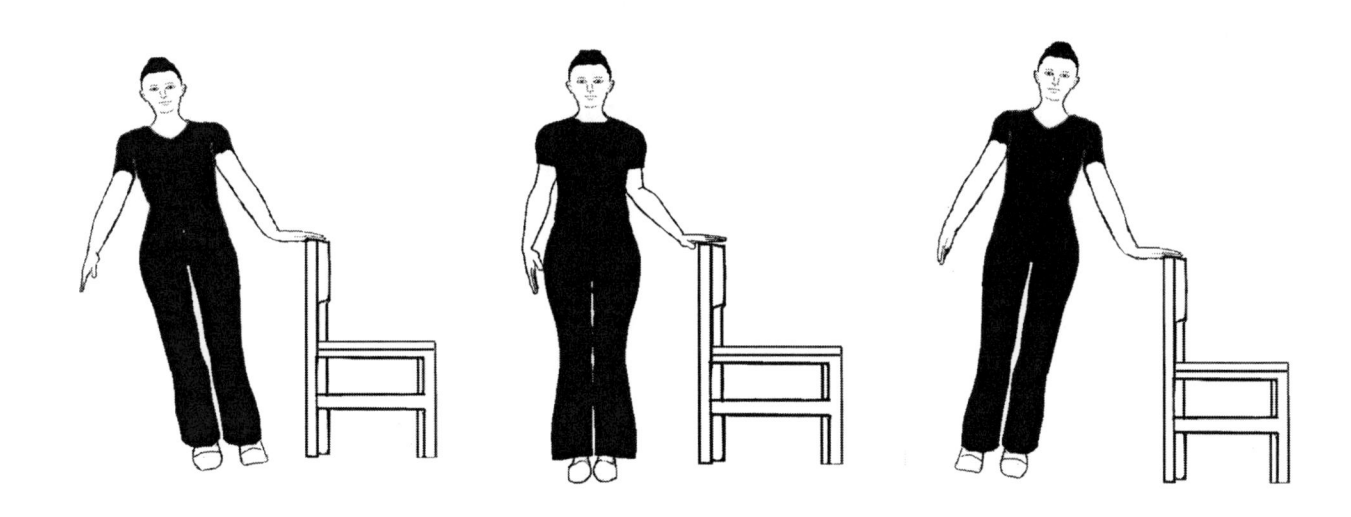

Warrior I Pose

Check your posture before you begin. Keep your shoulders down and your knees slightly bent. Tuck in the chin and think about pushing the crown of the head up to the ceiling without lifting your chin. The abdominal muscles are lightly pulled in, but not so much that it restricts your breathing.

To start step your left leg back into a lunge position. Feet and toes should be pointing straight forward; do not turn your back foot or leg out to the side. Make sure that your right knee does not extend past your right ankle bone. You should be able to look down at your right knee and see both your right toes and the arch of the right foot. If you need a deeper stretch step the feet wider apart rather then lunging the right knee beyond the front toes. This will help to protect the knee joint from injury.

Lift the back heel off of the floor. Bring the hips under the shoulders, do not lean the upper body forward. Gently pull the right hip back, as you bring the left hip forward. Without lifting the shoulders, reach the arms out in front of you, with the palms facing each other.

Hold for five to ten deep belly breaths, or for as long as is comfortable Repeat on the left side.

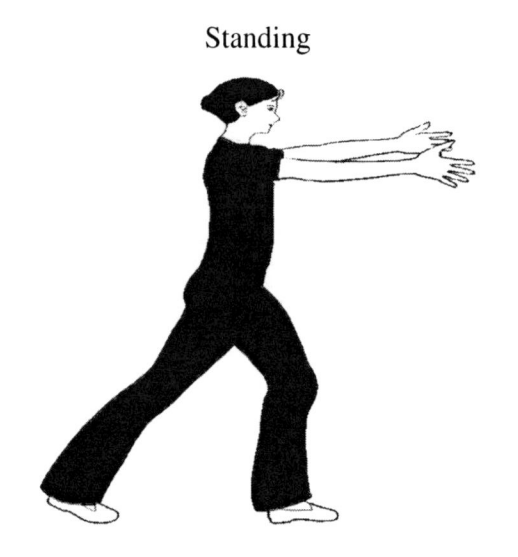

Standing

Standing with Assistance

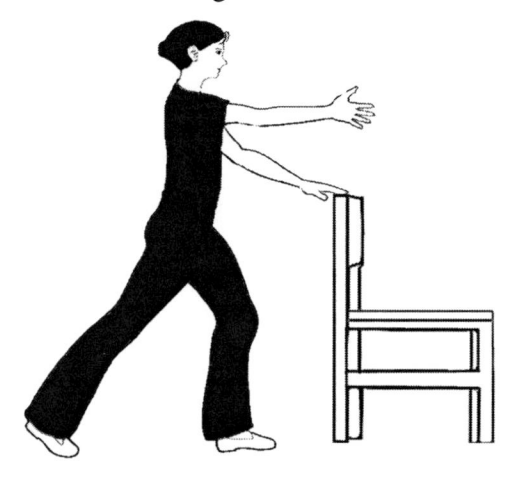

Seated

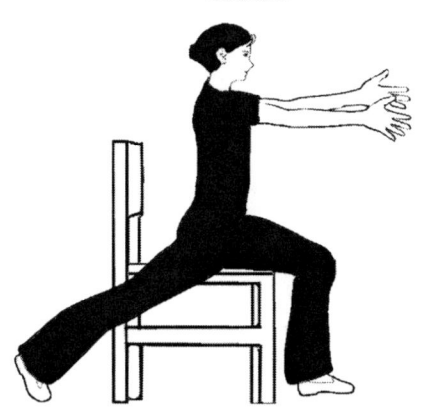

Checklist
- ✓ Stand or sit up straight, away from the back of the chair if possible
- ✓ Keep the spine straight and the shoulders over the hips
- ✓ Keep the shoulders down away from the ears
- ✓ Keep the natural curve in the low back
- ✓ Keep the front knee aligned over the front ankle
- ✓ Hold for five to ten deep belly breaths, or to comfort
- ✓ Use diaphragmatic breathing through the nose as much as possible
- ✓ Do not exercise to the point of strain or discomfort
- ✓ Remember the goal of yoga is to find that point where you are challenging yourself but not struggling

Warrior II Pose

Check your posture before you begin. Shoulders should be back and down and over the hips. Knees should remain slightly bent. The chin should be tucked in and push the crown of the head up to the ceiling without lifting your chin. Lightly contract the abdominal muscles, but not so much that it restricts your breathing.

Step your right foot out to the side into a lunge position. The back knee is straight, but not locked and the front knee is bent. Turn the toes of the left foot in, so the left foot is at about a 45-degree angle.

Turn the right toes out to the right side. Make sure that your right knee does not extend past your right ankle bone. You should be able to look down at your right knee and see both your right toes and the arch of the right foot.

Also check that your right knee is directly over your ankle and not rolling in or out. If you need a deeper stretch step the feet wider apart rather then lunging the right knee forward beyond the toes. This will help to protect the knee joint from injury.

Bring the arms out to the side about shoulder height with the palms facing the floor. Look out over your right hand. Bring the hips under the shoulders, do not lean the upper body forward.

Hold for five to ten deep belly breaths, or for as long as is comfortable. Repeat on the left side.

Standing

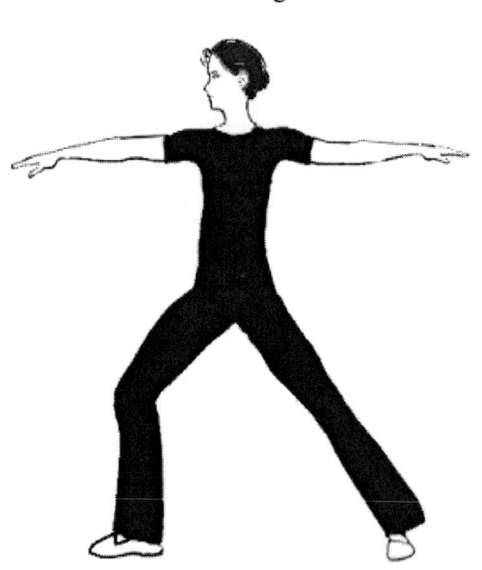

Standing with Assistance

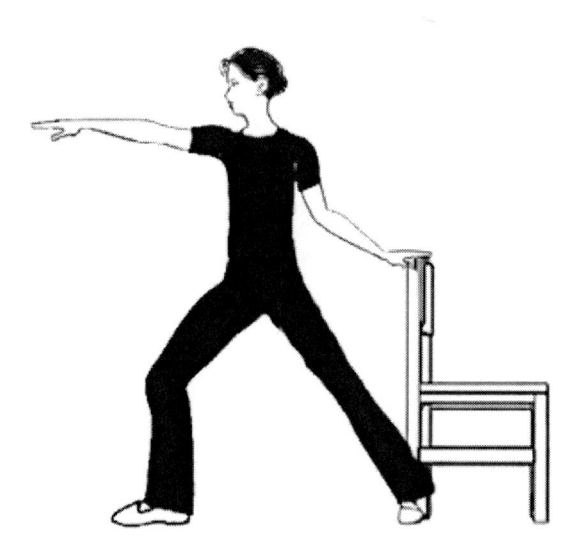

Seated

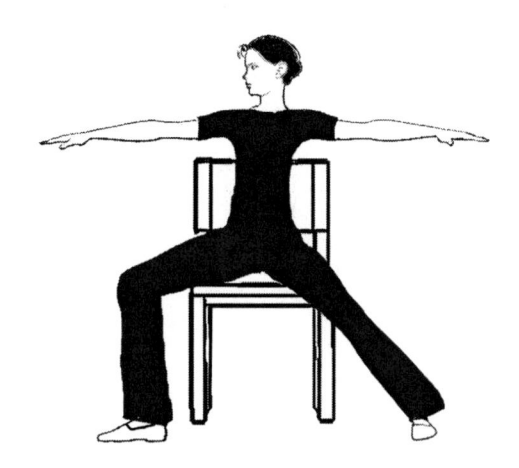

Checklist
- Stand or sit up straight, away from the back of the chair if possible
- Keep the spine straight and the shoulders over the hips
- Keep the shoulders down away from the ears
- Keep the natural curve in the low back
- Keep the front knee aligned over the front ankle
- Hold for five to ten deep belly breaths, or to comfort
- Use diaphragmatic breathing through the nose as much as possible
- Do not exercise to the point of strain or discomfort
- Remember the goal of yoga is to find that point where you are challenging yourself but not struggling

Lateral Angle Pose

    Check your posture before you begin. Shoulders should be back and down and over the hips. Knees should remain slightly bent. Tuck in the chin and think about pushing the crown of the head up to the ceiling without lifting your chin. The abdominal muscles are lightly pulled in, but not so much that it restricts your breathing.

    Step your right foot out to the side into a lunge position. The back knee is straight but not locked, and the front knee is bent.

    Turn the toes of the left foot in, so the foot is at about a forty-five degree angle.

    Turn the right toes out to the right side. Make sure that your right knee does not extend past your right ankle bone. You should be able to look down at your right knee and see both your right toes and the arch of the right foot.

    Also check that your right knee is directly over your ankle and not rolling in or out. If you need a deeper stretch step the feet wider apart rather then lunging the right knee forward beyond the toes. This will help to protect the knee joint from injury.

    Reach out to the right and bend at the waist, bringing your right hand (or for a deeper stretch your right elbow) to your right knee.

    Drop the left hip down making a straight line from your heel to your shoulder.

    Look up at your left hand if possible. If this is too strenuous just look straight ahead.

    Draw the left arm back to open the chest. Do not lean the upper body forward.

    If placing your hand on your knee is too deep of a stretch place your hand on the seat of a chair or for less stretch the back of the chair.

    Hold for five to ten deep belly breaths, or for as long as is comfortable. Repeat on the left side.

Standing

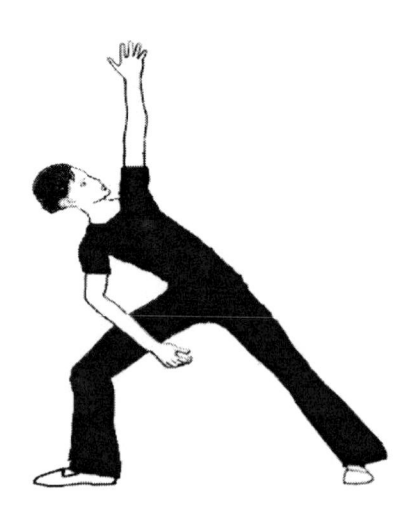

Standing with assistance

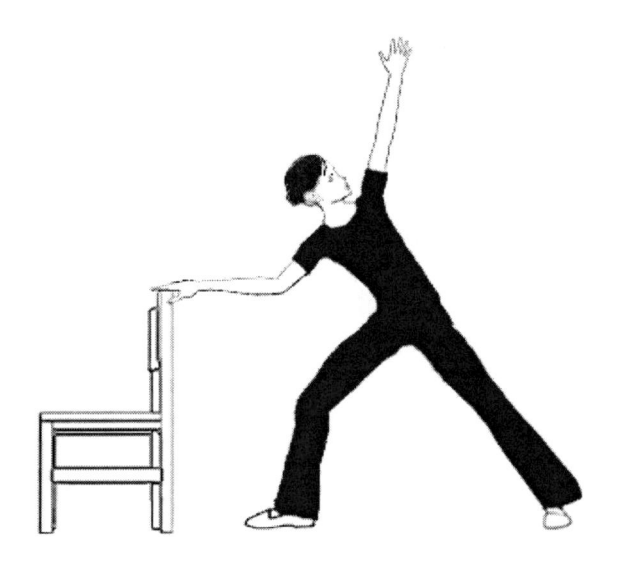

Placing the hand on the seat of the chair   Seated

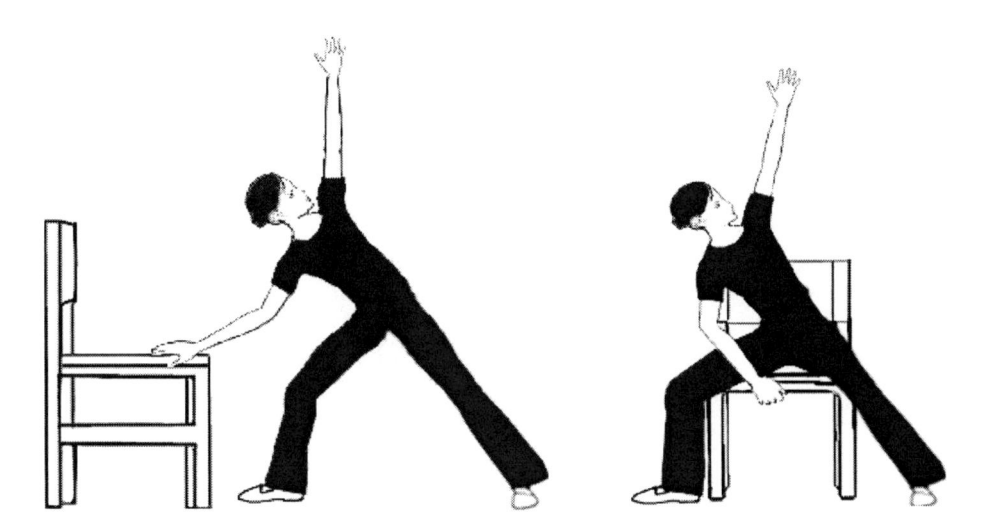

Checklist
- ✓ Keep the front knee aligned over the front ankle
- ✓ Do not tip the body forward, focus on rotating the bottom hip forward and the top shoulder back
- ✓ Hold for five to ten deep belly breaths, or to comfort
- ✓ Use diaphragmatic breathing through the nose as much as possible
- ✓ Remember the goal of yoga is to find that point where you are challenging yourself but not struggling

Chair Pose

This posture is only shown standing, as there is no comparable seated version. If you are unable to do standing work, skip ahead to the next page. Check your posture before you begin. Shoulders should be back and down and over the hips. Tuck in the chin and think about pushing the crown of the head up to the ceiling without lifting your chin. The abdominal muscles are lightly pulled in, but not so much that it restricts your breathing.

Without lifting the shoulders up, raise your arms out in front of you shoulder height, palms facing down. Begin to bend the knees, reaching the buttocks back as if you were about to sit in a chair.

Keep your weight forward in your toes to avoid falling backwards. You should feel this posture in the thigh muscles, not the knee joints. The closer the feet are together, the more challenging this posture is. If you feel unsteady, step the feet wider apart, or to challenge yourself, bring the feet together. Go as low as you can without causing discomfort in the knees, but do not let the buttocks go below the knees. Only go as low as you would to sit in a chair. *If you tend to fall backwards, place a chair behind you for safety.* Keep the natural curve in the low back.

Hold for five to ten deep belly breaths, or for as long as is comfortable.

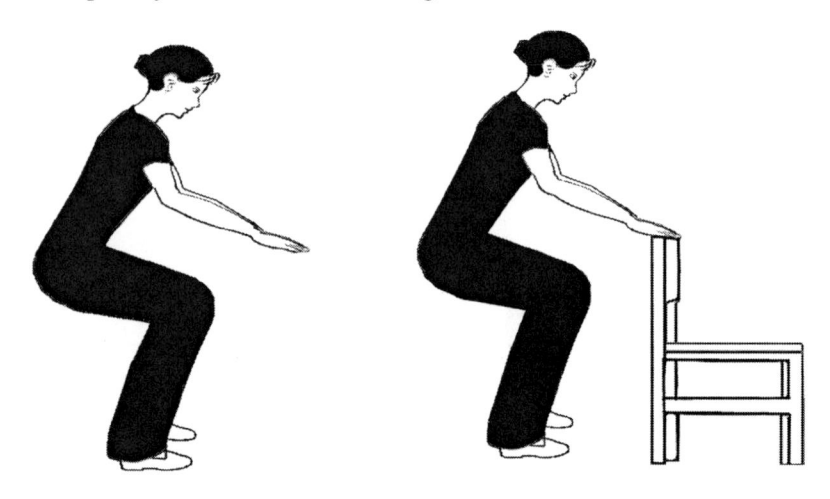

Checklist
- ✓ Only go as low as you can without knee discomfort
- ✓ Hold for five to ten deep belly breaths, or to comfort
- ✓ Keep the natural curve in the low back
- ✓ Use diaphragmatic breathing through the nose as much as possible
- ✓ Remember the goal of yoga is to find that point where you are challenging yourself but not struggling

Warrior III Pose

Check your posture before you begin. Shoulders are back and down and the knees should remain bent. Tuck in the chin and think about pushing the crown of the head up to the ceiling without lifting your chin. Lightly contract the abdominal muscles, but not so much that it restricts your breathing.

Without raising the shoulders up, bring your arms up in front of you about shoulder height with the palms facing each other.

Begin to lift the right leg up straight behind you. The shoulders can tip *slightly* forward, but keep the body in a straight line from the heel to the head.

Keep the natural curve in the low back. Lift the back leg as much as your balance allows.

Check that you do not lift the leg so high that you cause discomfort in the low back. The purpose of this posture is to challenge your ability to stand on one foot, and should not cause back pain.

The left knee (the leg you are standing on) should not be locked.

Hold for five to ten deep belly breaths, or for as long as is comfortable. Repeat on the left.

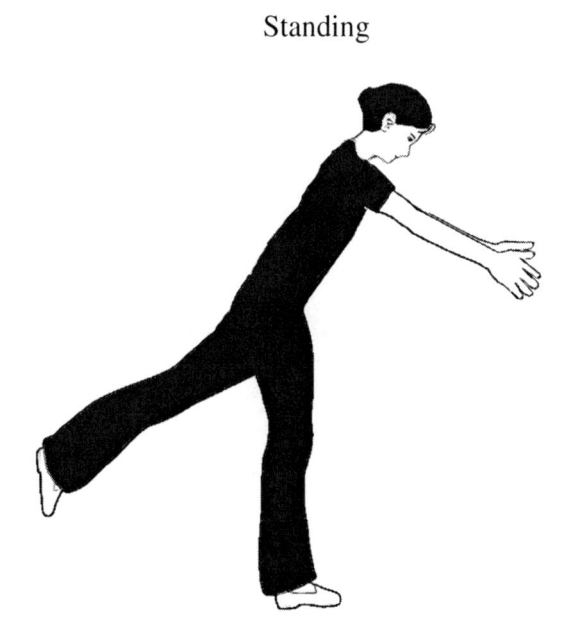

Standing

Standing with Assistance

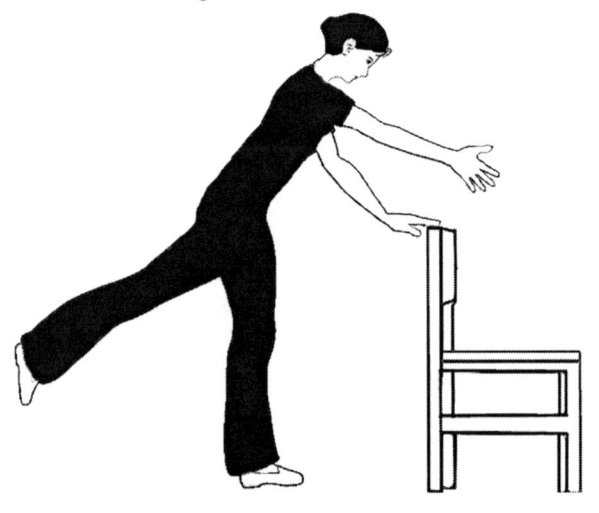

Seated

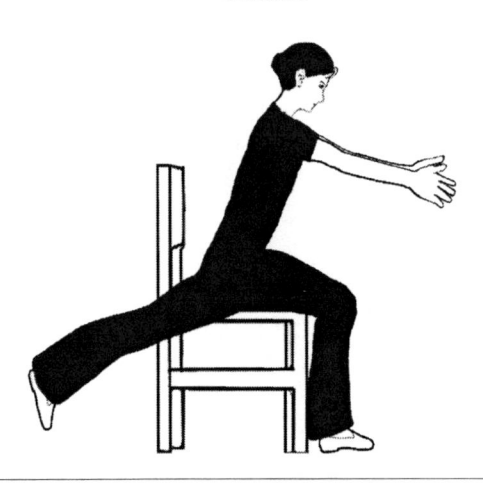

Checklist
- Keep the shoulders down away from the ears
- Keep the front knee bent, the back knee straight and the natural curve in the low back
- Keep the bent knee aligned over the ankle
- Do not lift the leg so high that you create back pain
- Hold for five to ten deep belly breaths, or to comfort
- Use diaphragmatic breathing through the nose as much as possible
- Remember the goal of yoga is to find that point where you are challenging yourself but not struggling

Tree Pose

Check your posture before you begin. Shoulders should be back and down and over the hips. Knees should remain slightly bent. Tuck in the chin and think about pushing the crown of the head up to the ceiling without lifting your chin. The abdominal muscles are lightly pulled in, but not so much that it restricts your breathing.

Without raising the shoulders up, lift your arms up overhead with the palms facing each other. Shift your weight to the left leg.

Bend the right knee and lift the right foot, placing the sole of the right foot against the inside of the left leg. The higher you lift the right foot, the more challenging this posture is. Do not place the right foot directly on the side of the left knee in order to protect the joint. If you find this too challenging you can start by keeping the right toes on the floor.

Bring the hips under the shoulders. Keep the natural curve in the low back. Lift the leg as high as your balance allows. The left knee (the leg you are standing on) should not be locked. Your right foot should be below or above the knee joint. Hold for five to ten deep belly breaths, or for as long as is comfortable. Repeat on the left.

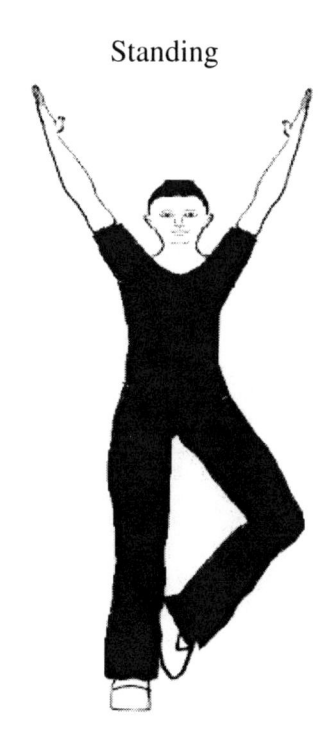

Standing

Standing with Assistance

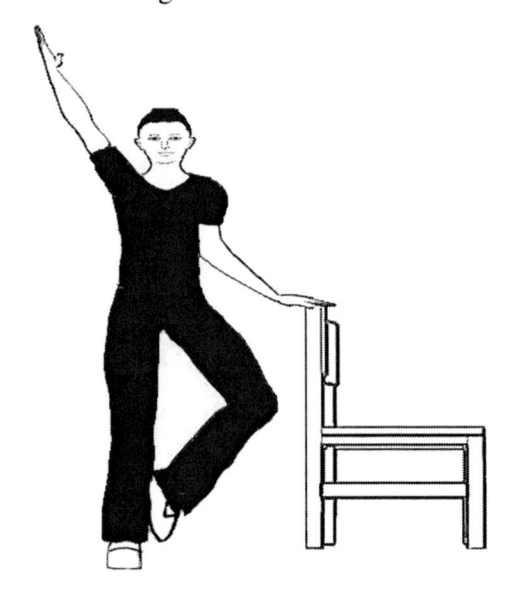

Seated

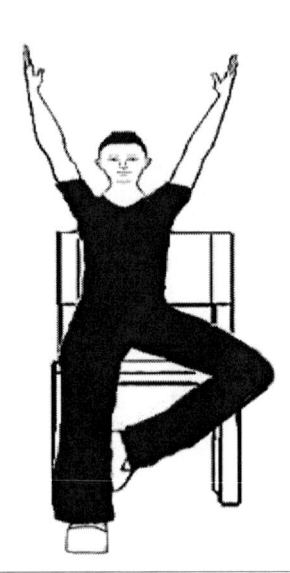

Checklist
- ✓ Stand or sit up straight and keep the shoulders down away from the ears
- ✓ Keep the hips under the shoulders
- ✓ Hold for five to ten deep belly breaths, or to comfort
- ✓ Use diaphragmatic breathing through the nose as much as possible
- ✓ Remember the goal of yoga is to find that point where you are challenging yourself but not struggling

Victory Squat Pose/W Stretch

Check your posture before you begin. Shoulders should be back and down and over the hips. Knees slightly bent. Tuck in the chin and think about pushing the crown of the head up to the ceiling without lifting your chin. The abdominal muscles are lightly pulled in, but not so much that it restricts your breathing.

Turn the feet out and step very wide apart. Bend the knees and come into a squat keeping the knees aligned over the ankles.

Only lower until you feel a stretch in the top of the thighs but not so low that it bothers your knees.

Without raising the shoulders up, bring the arms into a "W" keeping the hands in a straight line with the elbows.

Keep the natural curve in the low back. Keeping the hands, wrists and elbows in line, draw the arms back as far as you can, squeezing the shoulder blades together in the back. Do not let the head come forward. Hold for five to ten deep belly breaths, or to comfort.

Victory Squat

Victory Squat Back View

This exercise is helpful to correct a forward head posture. To check if your back is straight you can hold this posture with your back against a wall. Follow the above steps keeping the buttocks and back against the wall. If possible let the back of the head touch the wall, keeping the chin parallel to the floor. Do not tilt your head back to make it touch. If your head does not touch, just come back as far as you can. With consistent stretching you may eventually be able to go back further. Keeping the hands and elbows in line, draw the elbows and hands back as close to the wall as you can. Let the elbows and hands touch the wall, if you can do so without hurting your shoulders or arching your back. Hold for five to ten deep belly breaths, or to comfort.

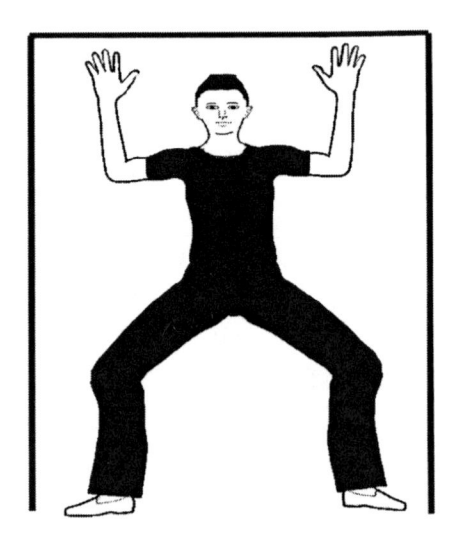

Against a Wall *Seated*

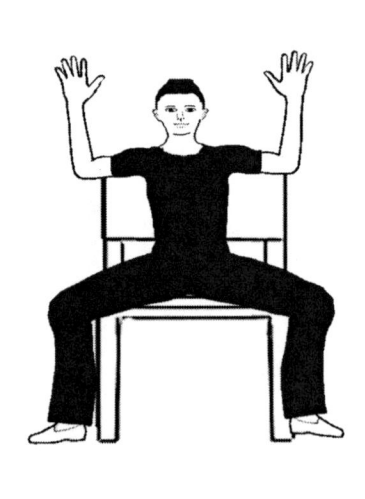

Checklist
- ✓ Stand or sit up straight and keep the shoulders down away from the ears
- ✓ Keep the hips under the shoulders and the natural curve in the low back
- ✓ Hold for five to ten deep belly breaths, or to comfort
- ✓ Use diaphragmatic breathing through the nose as much as possible
- ✓ Remember the goal of yoga is to find that point where you are challenging yourself but not struggling

Dancer's Pose/Quadriceps Stretch

Check your posture before you begin. Shoulders should be back and down and over the hips. Tuck in the chin and think about pushing the crown of the head up to the ceiling without lifting your chin. The abdominal muscles are lightly pulled in, but not so much that it restricts your breathing.

Shift your weight into the left leg. Bend the right knee, bringing the heel as close to the buttocks as you can. Bring the hips under the shoulders. Bring the knees together and let the right knee point down towards the floor as much as possible.

If it is comfortable to do so, hold onto your right ankle, sock or pant leg. If this is creates too deep of a stretch just lift the heel back. Hold for five to ten deep belly breaths, or for as long as is comfortable. Repeat on the left.

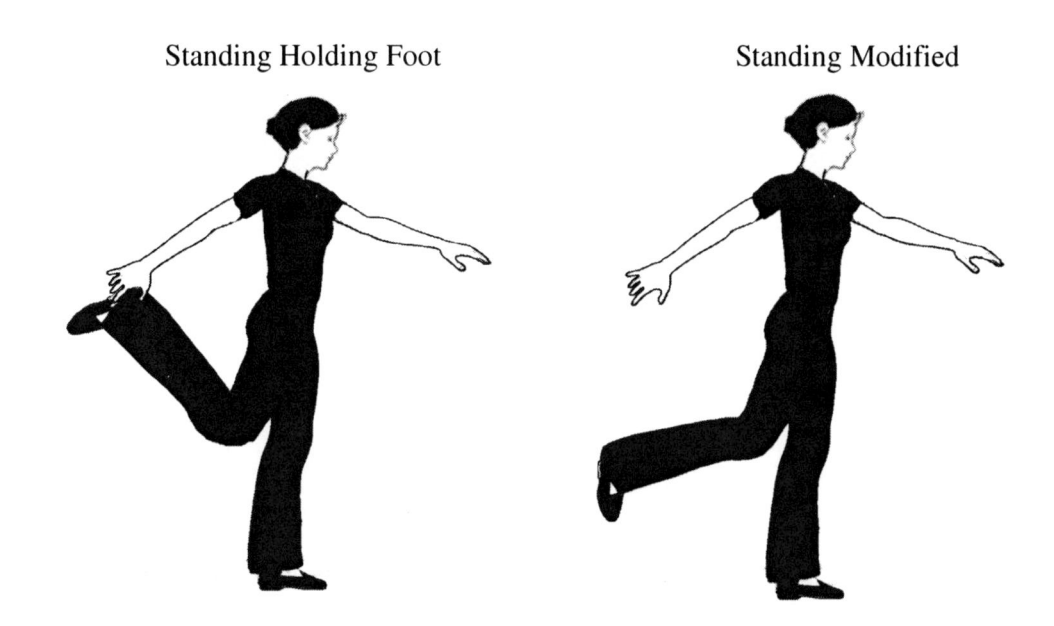

Standing Holding Foot

Standing Modified

Standing with assistance

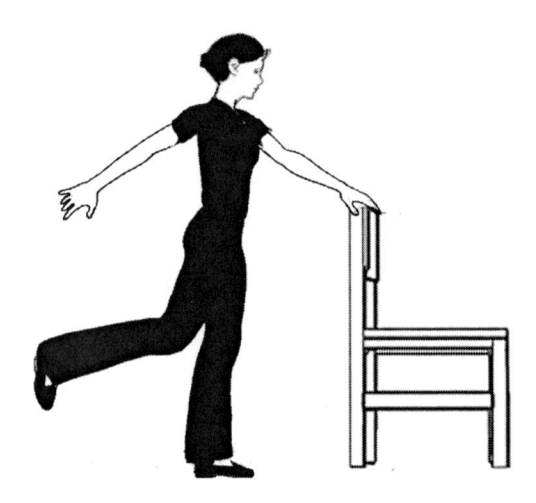

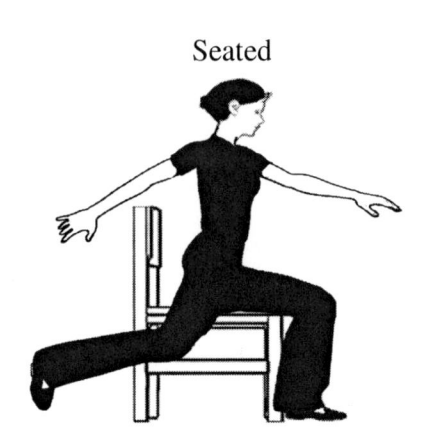

Seated

Checklist
- ✓ Stand or sit up straight
- ✓ Keep the shoulders down away from the ears
- ✓ Keep the hips under the shoulder
- ✓ Keep the knees slightly bent and the natural curve in the low back
- ✓ Hold for five to ten deep belly breaths, or to comfort
- ✓ Use diaphragmatic breathing through the nose as much as possible
- ✓ Remember the goal of yoga is to find that point where you are challenging yourself but not struggling

Hamstring Stretch/Seated Forward Bend Pose

Check your posture before you begin. Keep the shoulders down and knees slightly bent. Tuck in the chin and think about pushing the crown of the head up to the ceiling without lifting your chin. Lightly contract the abdominal muscles, but not so much that it restricts your breathing.

Step your right foot forward into a lunge position. The back knee is straight but not locked, and the front knee is bent.

Both feet and toes are facing forward. Make sure that your right knee does not extend past your right ankle bone. You should be able to look down at your right knee and see both your right toes and the arch of the right foot.

If you need a deeper stretch step the feet wider apart rather then lunging the right knee beyond the toes. This will help to protect the knee joint from injury.

Bring the hips under the shoulders. Press your back heel down to the floor, but be careful to not lock the back knee. Hold for five to ten deep belly breaths, or for as long as is comfortable. Repeat with the right leg back.

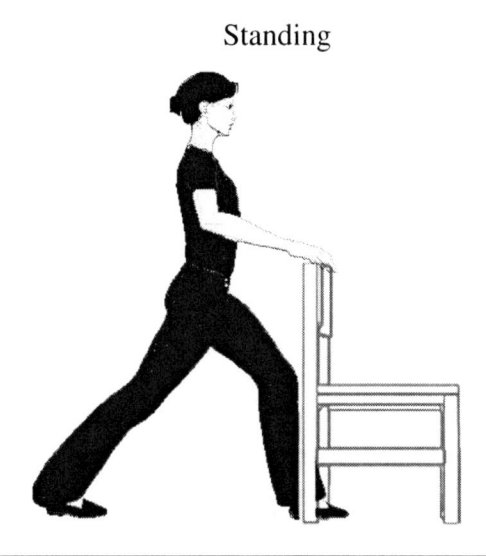

Standing

Checklist
- ✓ Stand up straight
- ✓ Keep the shoulders down away from the ears
- ✓ Keep the hips under the shoulders
- ✓ Make sure both feet point forward and do not turn the feet out
- ✓ Keep the knees slightly bent and the natural curve in the low back
- ✓ Hold for five to ten deep belly breaths, or to comfort
- ✓ Use diaphragmatic breathing through the nose as much as possible
- ✓ Remember the goal of yoga is to find that point where you are challenging yourself but not struggling

Seated

Sit at the front edge of the chair. Extend your right leg forward and pull the toes towards you. Keep the back straight and bring your chest forward, hinging at the hips. Do not round your back or slump forward.

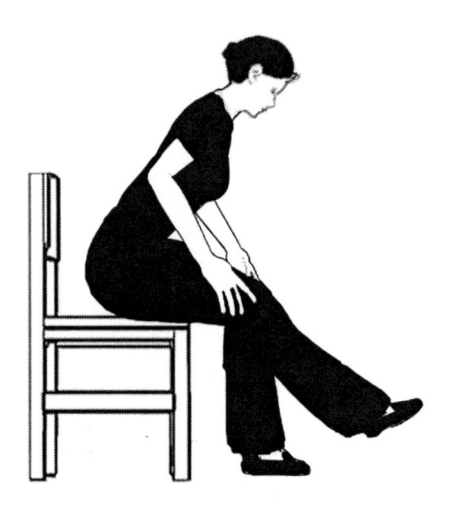

Checklist
✓ Sit up straight
✓ Keep the shoulders down away from the ears
✓ Keep the hips under the shoulders
✓ Keep the knees slightly bent and the natural curve in the low back
✓ Hold for five to ten deep belly breaths, or to comfort
✓ Use diaphragmatic breathing through the nose as much as possible
✓ Do not exercise to the point of strain or discomfort
✓ Remember the goal of yoga is to find that point where you are challenging yourself but not struggling

Seated Half Lotus Pose/Hip Stretch

Check your posture before you begin. Shoulders should be back and down and over the hips. Tuck in the chin and think about pushing the crown of the head up to the ceiling without lifting your chin. The abdominal muscles are lightly pulled in, but not so much that it restricts your breathing.

Use caution with this exercise if you have had a hip replacement or have significant hip pain. If you have had a hip replacement, check with your health care provider about the appropriateness of this stretch. If in doubt follow the instructions for the modification.

Sit up straight. For this stretch you may wish to sit against the back of the chair to support your back. Bring your right ankle bone up to the left knee. Let the right knee drop out to the side as much as possible. Make sure that you are not just crossing the legs. It should be your right ankle bone on your left knee, not your right knee. Hold for five to ten deep belly breaths, or for as long as is comfortable. Repeat with the left leg. *Modification:* Cross your right ankle over your left ankle and let the knee fall out to the side as much as possible. Then repeat with the left ankle over the right.

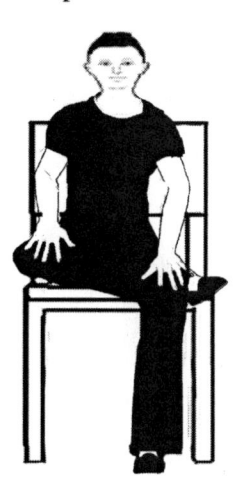

Hip Stretch   Hip Stretch Modified

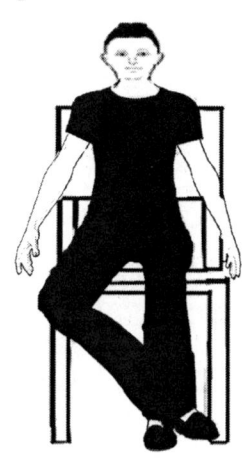

	Checklist
✓	Sit up straight and keep the shoulders down away from the ears
✓	Check that you are not crossing the legs
✓	Hold for five to ten deep belly breaths, or to comfort
✓	Use diaphragmatic breathing through the nose as much as possible
✓	Do not exercise to the point of strain or discomfort
✓	Remember the goal of yoga is to find that point where you are challenging yourself but not struggling

Seated Spinal Twist Pose

Check your posture before you begin. Shoulders should be back and down and over the hips. Tuck in the chin and think about pushing the crown of the head up to the ceiling without lifting your chin. The abdominal muscles are lightly pulled in, but not so much that it restricts your breathing.

Use caution with this posture if you have any sensitivities in the back. Check with your health care provider if you have concerns about the appropriateness of twisting movements.

Sit up straight away from the back of the chair if possible. Reach the left hand to the outside of the right knee. Turn to the right beginning the movement at the waist. Reach your right arm back behind you and look over your right shoulder. Turn as far as you comfortably can and look behind you as far as you can. You can press *gently* against your knee to help you twist further. Each time you inhale sit up straighter. Each time you exhale turn from the waist a little bit more. Hold for five to ten deep belly breaths, or for as long as is comfortable. Repeat with the right hand on the outside of the left knee.

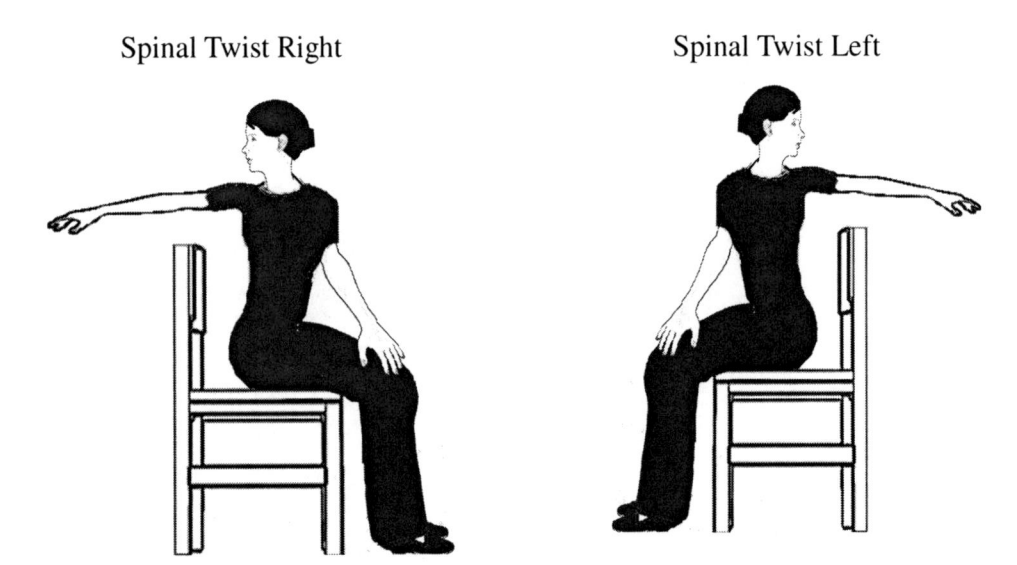

Spinal Twist Right   Spinal Twist Left

Checklist
- ✓ Sit up straight and away from the back of the chair as much as possible
- ✓ Keep the shoulders down away from the ears
- ✓ Keep the natural curve in the low back
- ✓ Use caution if you have back sensitivities
- ✓ Hold for five to ten deep belly breaths, or to comfort
- ✓ Use diaphragmatic breathing through the nose as much as possible
- ✓ Do not exercise to the point of strain or discomfort
- ✓ Remember the goal of yoga is to find that point where you are challenging yourself but not struggling

Knee To Chest Pose

Sit towards the front edge of the chair and lean your upper back against the chair. Keep the abdominal muscles contracted to help protect your back.

Draw your right knee up towards your chest and if possible hold underneath the knee. Be careful not to hold in front of the knee as this will compress the joint. If your hands will not reach under your right knee, you can wrap a towel or strap under the foot and hold the ends with your hands. Hold for five to ten deep belly breaths, or for as long as is comfortable. Repeat with the left knee.

Knee To Chest Sit   Knee To Chest Sit With Towel

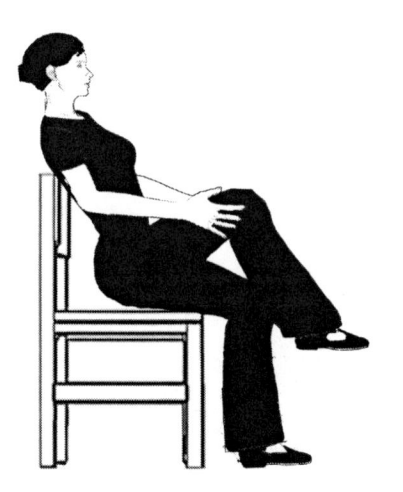

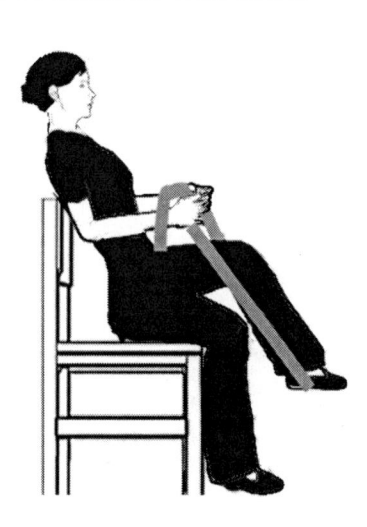

Checklist
✓ Keep the shoulders down away from the ears
✓ Keep the natural curve in the low back
✓ Make sure you hold on underneath the knee, not in front of the knee
✓ Hold for five to ten deep belly breaths, or to comfort
✓ Use diaphragmatic breathing through the nose as much as possible
✓ Do not exercise to the point of strain or discomfort
✓ Remember the goal of yoga is to find that point where you are challenging yourself but not struggling

Ankle Exercises

Check your posture before you begin. Shoulders should be back and down and over the hips. Tuck in the chin and think about pushing the crown of the head up to the ceiling without lifting your chin. The abdominal muscles are lightly pulled in, but not so much that it restricts your breathing.

Plantar and Dorsi Flexion

Sit up straight and away from the back of the chair if possible. Lift the right foot slightly off the floor. Point the toes of the right foot down, pressing through the ball of the foot. Then pull the toes back towards you, pressing out through the heel. Repeat eight to twelve times taking deep belly breaths. Repeat with the left foot.

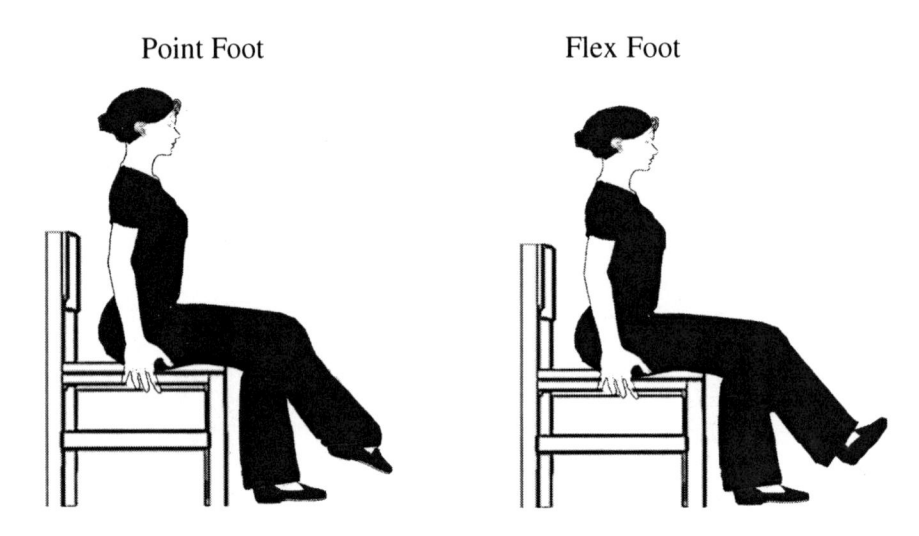

Point Foot Flex Foot

Ankle Circles

Sit up straight and away from the back of the chair if possible. Lift the right foot slightly off the floor. Circle the ankle in one direction, and then the other. Be careful to circle just the ankle and not the whole leg. Repeat eight to twelve times each way, taking deep belly breaths. Repeat with the left foot.

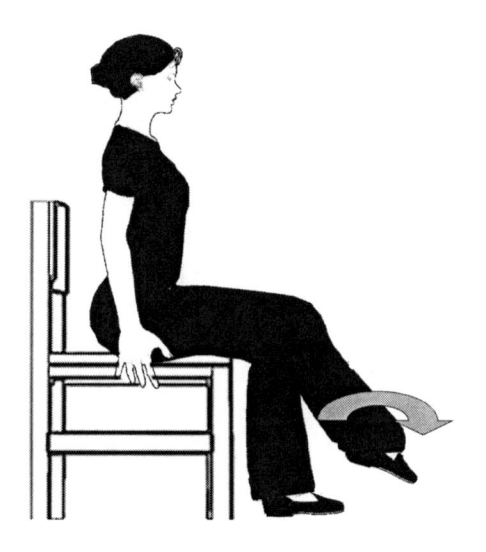

Checklist
- ✓ Sit up straight and away from the back of the chair as much as possible
- ✓ Keep the shoulders down away from the ears
- ✓ Keep the natural curve in the low back
- ✓ Make sure you move just the ankle and not the whole leg
- ✓ Use diaphragmatic breathing through the nose as much as possible
- ✓ Do not exercise to the point of strain or discomfort
- ✓ Remember the goal of yoga is to find that point where you are challenging yourself but not struggling

Floor Exercises

On days when you feel able floor exercises can be very beneficial. The floor is a solid surface that provides feedback as to whether or not the back is straight and allows you to stretch deeply as you do not have to worry about falling. Doing floor exercises also keeps you in the habit of getting up and down. You may find that you will be able to get up more easily after a fall if you have been practicing getting up from the floor. Please refer to pages 42 through 45 for instructions as to how to get up and down safely. Performing these exercises on a couch or bed is not as beneficial as these surfaces are often too soft and do not provide enough support, however as always listen to your body and do what is best for you.

When performing floor exercises it is essential to maintain a pelvic tilt in the back in order to protect the back from injury. Letting your back arch off the floor can lead to back strain. It is also very important to keep your neck straight and in correct alignment. Make sure that the head does not tip backwards in order for your head to touch. This can place a lot of strain on the neck. To prevent neck strain place a towel or pillow under the head so the neck remains straight. However, do not use too high of a pillow as that will push the head forward. It is best to have someone help you get set up the first time so they can see if your neck is straight and to help you decide how much cushioning you need under your head.

Incorrect. Head tipped back

Incorrect. Too much support Head pushed forward

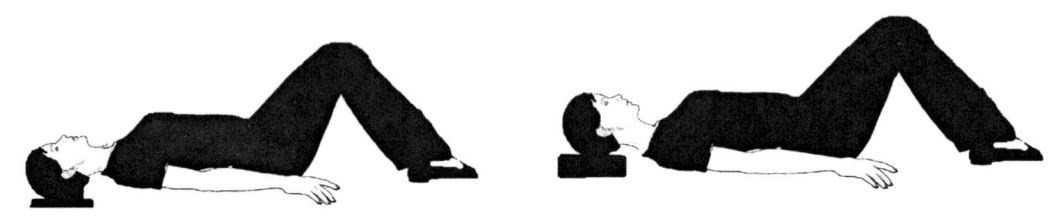

Correct Neck is straight and in alignment

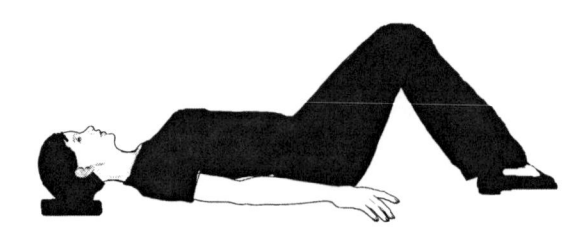

Pelvic Tilts

Lie on the floor on your back with the knees bent, feet on the floor. Make sure you keep the head and neck level, do not arch the head or tip the chin back. If you find that you are arching your neck, place a pillow under the head.

This exercise helps to strengthen the abdominal muscles and should be used with every floor exercise in order to protect the back from injury. Without lifting the hips or buttocks, press your low back down into the floor. Try to slip your hands under your low back. If you are doing this exercise correctly you should feel your low back tight against the floor, and you should be unable to get your hands under your back. Hold for a slow count of five. Then relax and let the low back arch enough so that you can slip your hands under your back. Repeat eight to twelve times.

Pelvic Tilt Down   Pelvic Tilt Arch

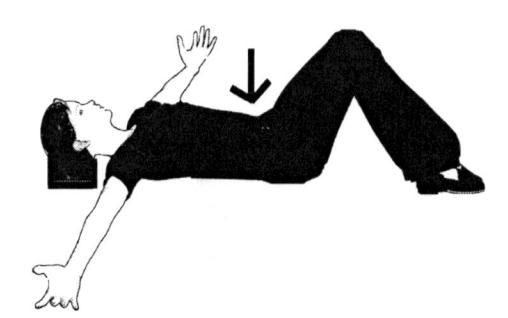

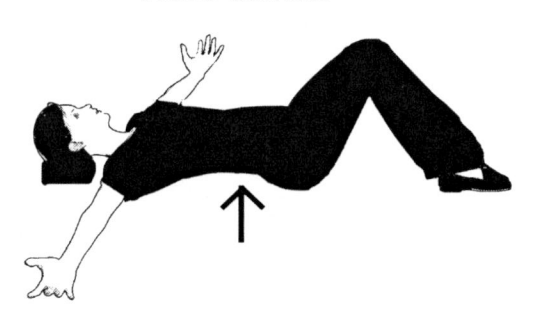

Checklist
✓ Make sure you keep your head and chin level
✓ Make sure you are moving the just the low back and not lifting the hips or buttocks
✓ Use diaphragmatic breathing through the nose as much as possible
✓ Do not exercise to the point of strain or discomfort
✓ Remember the goal of yoga is to find that point where you are challenging yourself but not struggling

Knee To Chest Pose

Lie on the floor on your back. Keep the head and neck level. If you find that you are arching your neck, place a pillow under the head. Begin with a pelvic tilt (pg. 161). Throughout this exercise make sure your low back stays in contact with the floor.

Without arching the back bring your right knee towards your chest. You can either hold the knee with your hands or wrap a towel or yoga strap around the knee and hold the ends of the strap with your hands. When holding the knee make sure you hold under the knee and not on top of the knee so you do not compress the joint. Make sure your head stays on the floor or pillow.

Do not hold the head off the floor just to reach your knee as this strains the neck. *Do not pull the leg in hard, just bring the knee in enough until you feel a gentle stretch in the back of the leg you are holding up.* Hold for five to ten deep belly breaths or for as long as is comfortable. Repeat with the other leg.

Knee To Chest On Floor   Knee To Chest With Towel On Floor

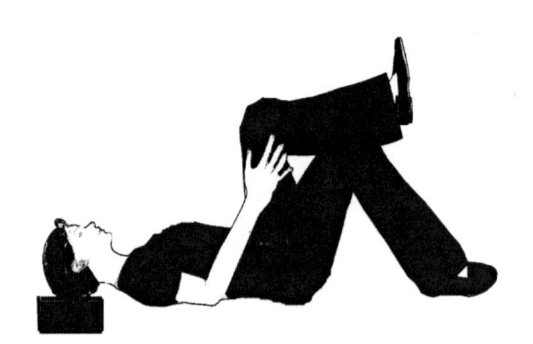

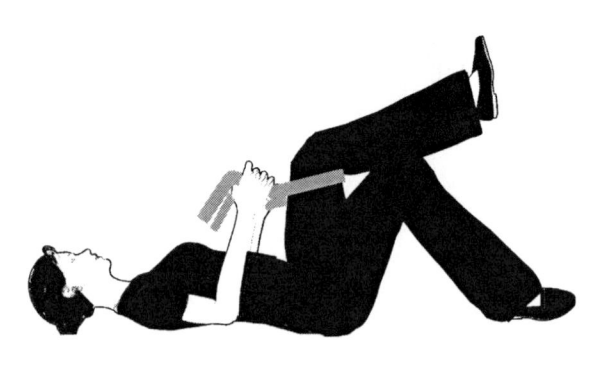

Checklist
- ✓ Make sure you keep your head and chin level and your head on the floor or pillow
- ✓ Make sure you keep the low back in contact with the floor
- ✓ Make sure you hold underneath the knee and not on top to avoid compressing the knee joint
- ✓ Use diaphragmatic breathing through the nose as much as possible
- ✓ Hold for five to ten deep belly breaths, or to comfort
- ✓ Do not exercise to the point of strain or discomfort
- ✓ Remember the goal of yoga is to find that point where you are challenging yourself but not struggling

Bridge

Lie on the floor on your back with the knees bent, feet on the floor. Make sure you keep the head and neck level do not arch the head or tip the chin back. If you find that you are arching your neck, place a pillow under the head. Tighten the buttocks muscles and lift the hips off the floor as high as you can. Make sure you do not let the head tip back as you lift, keep the neck straight and the chin level. Keep both knees pointing straight up to the ceiling do not let the knees roll in or out.

Exhale as you lift the hips and inhale as you lower the hips. Repeat eight to twelve times. After completing eight to twelve repetitions hold for a stretch in the lifted position for five to ten deep belly breaths, or for as long as is comfortable.

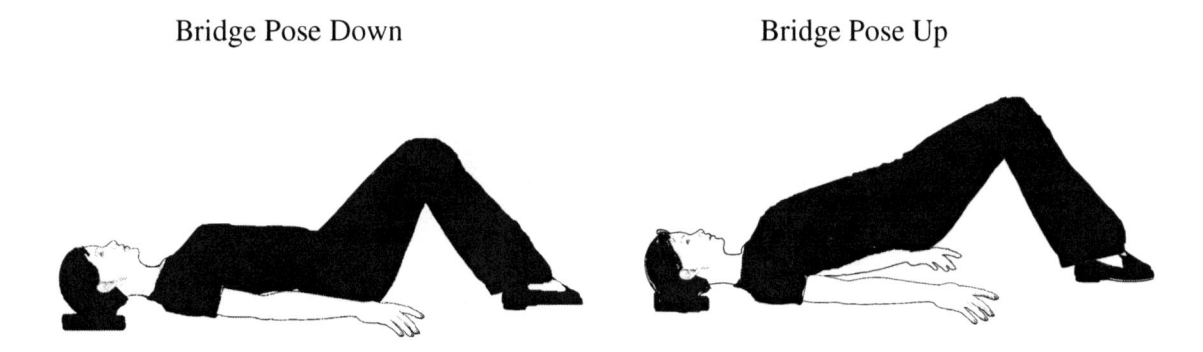

Bridge Pose Down   Bridge Pose Up

Checklist
✓ Make sure you keep your head and chin level
✓ Make sure you do not tip the head back when you lift the hips
✓ Keep the knees pointing up to the ceiling
✓ Use diaphragmatic breathing through the nose as much as possible
✓ Do not exercise to the point of strain or discomfort
✓ Remember the goal of yoga is to find that point where you are challenging yourself but not struggling

Supine Overhead Arm Reach

Lie on the floor on your back with the knees bent, feet on the floor. Make sure you keep the head and neck level using a pillow if necessary. Begin with a pelvic tilt.
Throughout this exercise make sure your low back stays in contact with the floor. Do not let the low back arch. If you are dealing with shoulder injuries use caution with the next two postures.
 Keeping the low back tight against the floor bring your right arm overhead with the palm facing up. Bring your arm as close as you can to the floor keeping your low back pressed into the floor. Keep the elbow close to the ear when the arm is back. If the back begins to arch make the movement smaller. The further away from the floor that your arm is the easier it is to keep your back flat. You will find that as your abdominal muscles strengthen and your shoulders become more flexible you will be able to lower your arm closer to the floor. Then bring the arm back and repeat with the left arm. Do eight to twelve repetitions. One repetition involves going to both sides.

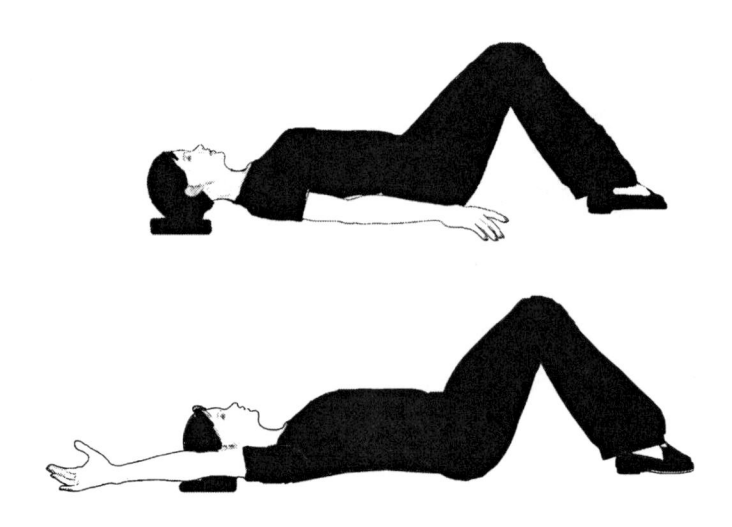

Checklist
- ✓ Make sure you keep your head and chin level
- ✓ Make sure you keep the low back in contact with the floor
- ✓ Use diaphragmatic breathing through the nose as much as possible
- ✓ Do not exercise to the point of strain or discomfort
- ✓ Remember the goal of yoga is to find that point where you are challenging yourself but not struggling

Supine Overhead Double Arm Reach

After completing eight to twelve repetitions reach both arms up straight. Clasp your hands and slowly bring your arms as close as you can to the floor keeping your low back pressed into the floor. Keep the elbows close to the ears when the arms are back. Then slowly lift the arms back up. If the back begins to arch make the movement smaller. Do eight to twelve repetitions. After completing eight to twelve repetitions hold for a stretch with both arms back and the back flat on the floor. Hold for five to ten deep belly breaths, or to comfort.

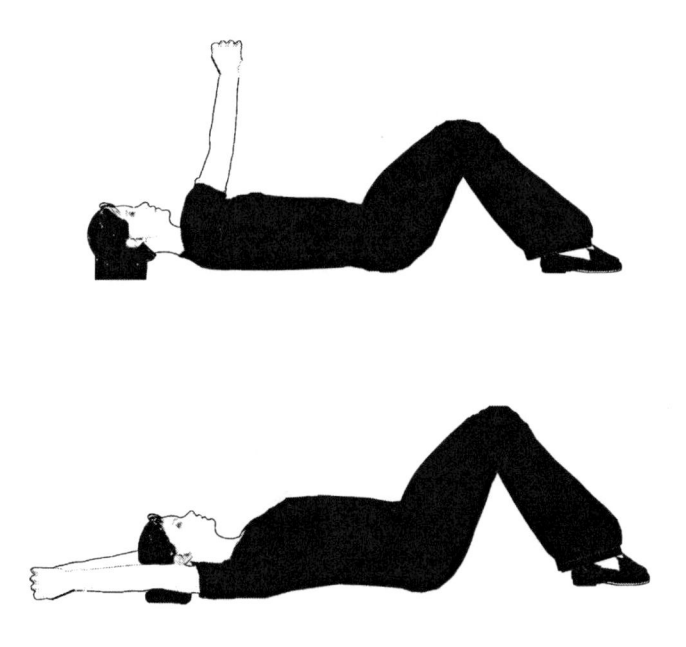

Checklist
- ✓ Make sure you keep your head and chin level
- ✓ Make sure you keep the low back in contact with the floor
- ✓ Use diaphragmatic breathing through the nose as much as possible
- ✓ Do not exercise to the point of strain or discomfort
- ✓ Remember the goal of yoga is to find that point where you are challenging yourself but not struggling

Supine Leg Lift

Lie on the floor on your back with the knees bent, feet on the floor. Make sure you keep the head and neck level do not arch the head or tip the chin back. If you find that you are arching your neck, place a pillow under the head. Begin with a pelvic tilt.
Throughout this exercise make sure your low back stays in contact with the floor. Do not let the low back arch. Keeping the low back tight against the floor lift your right leg straight up. Tighten your abdominal muscles and slowly, with control lower your leg as close as you can to the floor keeping your low back pressed into the floor. Then slowly lift the leg back up. If the back begins to arch make the movement smaller. The further away from the floor that your leg is the easier it is to keep your back flat. *Make sure you keep the left knee bent and the left foot on the floor. Stretching your left leg out along the floor can cause back strain.* You will find that as your abdominal muscles strengthen you will be able to lower your leg closer to the floor. Do eight to twelve repetitions and repeat with the left leg.

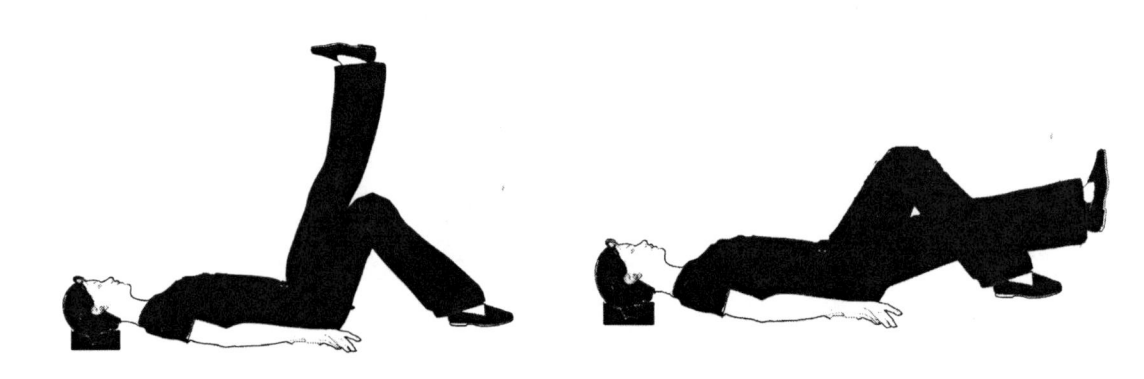

Checklist
- ✓ Make sure you keep your head and chin level
- ✓ Make sure you keep the low back in contact with the floor
- ✓ Keep the leg that is not moving bent with the foot on the floor. To prevent back injury avoid straightening both legs at the same time
- ✓ Use diaphragmatic breathing through the nose as much as possible
- ✓ Do not exercise to the point of strain or discomfort
- ✓ Remember the goal of yoga is to find that point where you are challenging yourself but not struggling

Supine Opposite Arm To Leg Reach

Lie on the floor on your back with the knees bent, feet on the floor. Keep the head and neck level using a pillow if necessary. Begin with a pelvic tilt. Throughout this exercise make sure your low back stays in contact with the floor. Do not let the low back arch.

Keeping the low back tight against the floor bring your right arm overhead and stretch your left leg out straight. Keep your right knee bent and the right foot on the floor. Bring your arm and leg as close as you can to the floor keeping your low back pressed into the floor. If the back begins to arch make the movement smaller. The further away from the floor that your arm and leg is, the easier it is to keep your back flat. You will find that as your abdominal muscles strengthen you will be able to lower your arm and leg closer to the floor.

Then bring the arm and leg all the way back. Repeat with the left arm and right leg. Keep the left knee bent and the left foot on the floor. Do eight to twelve repetitions. One repetition involves going to both sides.

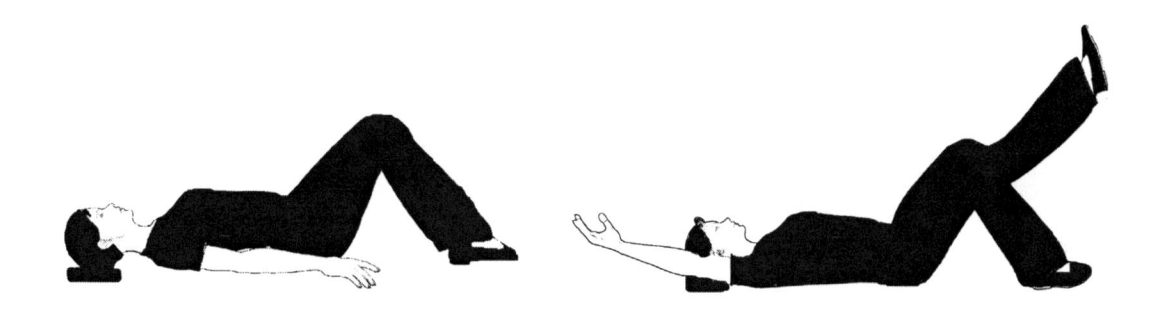

Checklist
- ✓ Make sure you keep your head and chin level
- ✓ Make sure you keep the low back in contact with the floor
- ✓ Keep the foot that is not moving flat on the floor. To avoid back injury do not lift both feet or arms off the floor at the same time.
- ✓ Use diaphragmatic breathing through the nose as much as possible
- ✓ Do not exercise to the point of strain or discomfort
- ✓ Remember the goal of yoga is to find that point where you are challenging yourself but not struggling

Hamstring Stretch

Keeping the low back tight against the floor bring your right knee towards your chest. Then straighten the leg, flex the foot, and press the heel up towards the ceiling. Straighten the leg as much as you can but do not lock the knee. If this bothers your low back you can also leave a soft bend in the knee. You can either leave your hands by your sides on the floor or wrap a towel or yoga strap around the foot and hold the ends of the towel or strap with your hands. Make sure your head stays on the floor or pillow. Do not hold the head off the floor as this strains the neck. Hold for five to ten deep belly breaths or for as long as is comfortable. Repeat with the other leg.

Hamstring Stretch Arms By Side On FloorHamstring Stretch Using a Towel On Floor

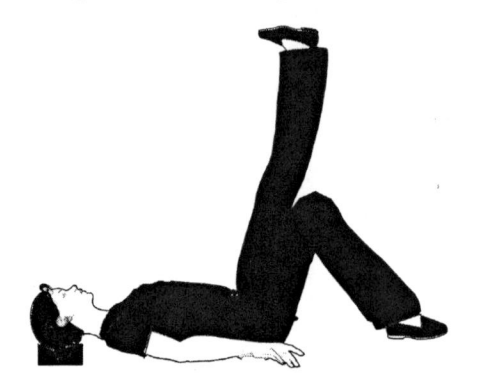

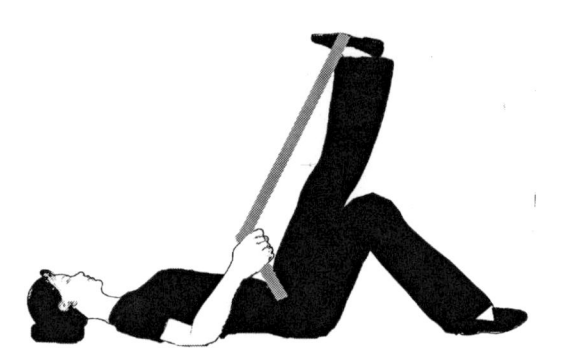

Checklist
- ✓ Make sure you keep your head and chin level and your head on the floor or pillow
- ✓ Make sure you keep the low back in contact with the floor
- ✓ The knee can be straight or have a soft bend, do not lock the knee
- ✓ Use diaphragmatic breathing through the nose as much as possible
- ✓ Hold for five to ten deep belly breaths
- ✓ Do not exercise to the point of strain or discomfort
- ✓ Remember the goal of yoga is to find that point where you are challenging yourself but not struggling

Spinal Twist

Be gentle with this movement if you have any back injuries. Lie on the floor on your back with the knees bent, feet on the floor. Make sure you keep the head and neck level do not arch the head or tip the chin back. If you find that you are arching your neck, place a pillow under the head.

Bring your arms out to the side in a "T" position with the palms facing the ceiling. Slowly lower both knees to one side. If it feels OK on your back you do not need to hold a pelvic tilt. You can let your left hip roll off the floor and let the knees come all the way to the floor. If that bothers your back stay in a pelvic tilt and do not drop the knees as far down. If comfortable you can turn your head and look away from your knees. Otherwise look straight up or towards your knees. Hold for five to ten deep belly breaths or for as long as is comfortable. Repeat other side.

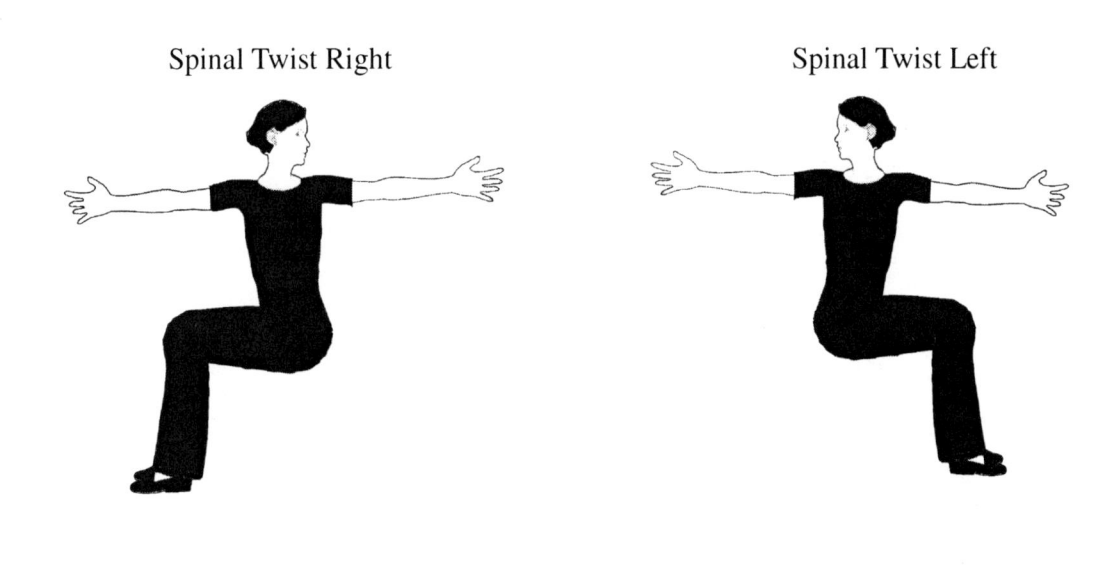

Spinal Twist Right

Spinal Twist Left

Checklist
- ✓ Make sure you keep your head and chin level and your head on the floor or pillow
- ✓ Only twist as far as it is comfortable to do so – use caution if your back is sensitive
- ✓ Use diaphragmatic breathing through the nose as much as possible
- ✓ Do not exercise to the point of strain or discomfort
- ✓ Remember the goal of yoga is to find that point where you are challenging yourself but not struggling

Bound Angle

The goal of this posture is to allow the body to completely relax. This posture is wonderful to open the shoulders and chest. You will need a yoga bolster or you can use a couch cushion or a pile of blankets and a few pillows.

If your neck is sensitive you can use the cushion the long way so that your head is supported. If your neck does not bother you, use the cushion the short way so that your neck and head come off the end of the cushion.

To get into this posture, sit up straight and place the bolster behind you, do not sit on it. Bring the soles of your feet together and let the knees drop out to the side. Place a pillow underneath each knee. The purpose of this posture is to let the whole body completely relax, so let the pillows support your knees if they do not reach the floor. Then, lie down over the cushion. If you are using the cushion the short way have the edge of it come just underneath your armpits so your shoulders are off the cushion.

The closer the heels are to the body the deeper the stretch, so adjust your heels accordingly. To support the neck you can also place a pillow or rolled up towel underneath the neck. Hold this posture for as long as feels comfortable. Take deep belly breaths into the chest and shoulders and let your body sink and rest into the cushions.

Bound Angle Bolster Short Way   Bound Angle Bolster Long Way

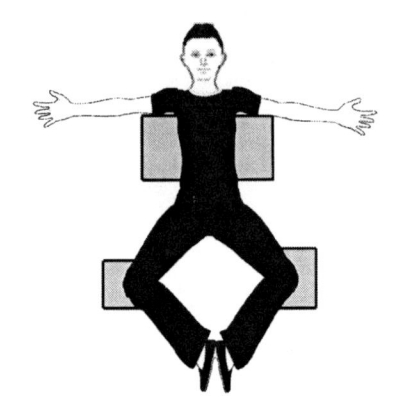

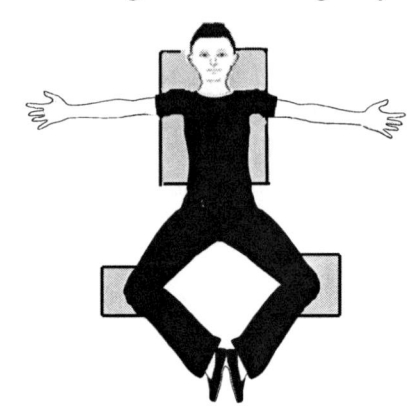

Checklist
- ✓ Use pillows to support the knees if they do not reach the floor to allow your leg muscles to fully relax
- ✓ Use diaphragmatic breathing through the nose as much as possible
- ✓ Do not exercise to the point of strain or discomfort
- ✓ Remember the goal of yoga is to find that point where you are challenging yourself but not struggling

Facial Exercises

Another common concern for those with Parkinson's disease is an absence of facial expression. Muscle rigidity in the face can produce a mask-like, staring appearance that can cause a person to lose the ability to use facial expressions when communicating with others. This decrease in the use of the facial muscles can also contribute to problems with eating and voice projection.

The following exercises help to strengthen the muscles of the face. It is helpful to practice these exercises in front of a mirror so you can see if you are doing the movements correctly. Perform each exercise once through and then go back to the first exercise and start again. Go through this sequence four to five times if you can. However just like any muscles in your body your facial muscles can become sore if overused so just do as much as you are able and build up slowly.

1) Pucker your lips in a kissing motion, and while in this puckered position try to bring the corners of your mouth together as close as possible.
2) Keeping your lips closed and teeth together. Smile as much as possible without opening your lips.
3) Keeping your lips closed, curl your lips into your mouth across your teeth.
4) Pout your lips, turning the bottom lip over.
5) Pretend you have just been exposed to a terrible smell. Wrinkle your nose and see how close you can bring your top lip to your nose.
6) With lips open and teeth apart, grin as widely as possible.
7) Frown as much as possible and try to bring your eyebrows over your eyes while pulling the eyebrows toward one another.
8) Show surprise. Lift your eyebrows up as far as possible while opening your eyes and mouth as far as possible.
9) While keeping your lips closed, make a chewing movement.
10) Open your mouth wide as possible. Separate your teeth by dropping your jaw and then push your jaw forward and back, and side to side.
11) Close the mouth and puff the cheeks with air, then purse the lips and blow the air out.

If you are having difficulty with speech, swallowing, eating or projecting your voice check into attending some Lee Silverman sessions with a therapist.
The sooner you start treatment the easier it is to correct any issues.
With a prescription from your doctor your sessions may be covered by insurance.

See the resources section for more information.

Voice Projection

Being able to project the voice so others can hear can often be difficult for those with Parkinson's disease. Some research suggests that speech problems occur in more than seventy percent of Parkinson's patients. Speech difficulty can be caused by rigidity of the facial muscles, loss of motor control, and impaired breathing ability. The tone of the voice can become monotonous, words may be repeated over and over, and the rate of speech may become very fast.

For those with Parkinson's disease the muscles needed for breathing and speech can become rigid and stiff and lose some of their elasticity. They can also become weak, making breathing and speaking very challenging. When the diaphragm and muscles in the chest wall become rigid, they do not expand completely when inhaling or relax completely during exhaling. It becomes more of a challenge to take a deep breath because the muscles do not move as easily. Shortness of breath also can occur from the stooped posture some Parkinson's patients experience, which leaves less space for the muscles to expand.

In addition, your exhaled air helps provide the power for the voice. Rigid muscles lead to a decreased ability to speak loudly enough because the muscles are not elastic and cannot move with variable force and speed. By strengthening your breathing muscles, you will get better voice volume and projection. The deep belly breathing technique used throughout this book can help to strengthen these muscles and help combat rigidity. The following exercises can also help you to better pronounce words and to project your voice.

1) The first step in improving voice projection is to practice the deep diaphragmatic (belly) breathing exercise introduced in the warm up and yoga chapters everyday. Just ten to fifteen minutes a day practicing this technique can improve lung capacity, overall energy levels and voice projection.

2) Recite the vowels and emphasize each one. Say them as loudly and clearly as you can. Take a deep breath in allowing the abdomen to expand. As you exhale, pull the abdomen in, push the air out and say the letter A as loud as you can. Repeat this process for all of the vowels.

3) Follow the same procedure but instead of saying the vowels as you exhale, say words like potato, or tomato. Focus on pushing the air and words out as loudly as you can and exaggerate the letters P and T.

4) Sing. Focus on taking deep breaths and pushing the words out. Singing is a great way to strengthen the lungs especially when combined with diaphragmatic breathing.

5) When speaking, break up long sentences by taking a breath. With Parkinson's disease the voice tends to get softer towards the end of the sentence. Try saying just a few words of a sentence and then stop. Then take a deep breath before saying the rest of the sentence.

Tai chi

Tai chi is a gentle low-impact traditional Chinese form of exercise that combines meditation and movement to improve and maintain health. It combines deep breathing with movements that flow slowly and smoothly from one to the other. The practice of Tai chi can help to enhance balance and body awareness and aid in making daily activities such as dressing walking, climbing, bending, and lifting easier.

Some of the principals of Tai chi are:

1) Energy (called chi) flows through the body along "energy pathways" called meridians. Illness may occur if the flow of chi is blocked or unbalanced at any point on these pathways. Tai chi is practiced to increase a person's chi energy and improve health through gentle, graceful, repeated movements.

2) Separate yin and yang. Nature including the body, consists of opposing forces called yin and yang and good health results when these forces are in balance. Tai chi movements are done in an attempt to help restore the body's balance of yin and yang. For example, if all of your weight is in your left leg then the left leg is yang and the unweighted right leg is yin. The goal is to become aware of this process.

3) Relaxation. The body should remain relaxed during Tai chi movements. The attention should be on continuously releasing tension especially in the neck, wrists, shoulders, and knees.

4) Turn from the waist. Eyes, nose and navel should turn as one unit.

5) The body is upright. As with all of the exercises in this book use good posture. The head remains upright. Think about lifting the crown of the head to the ceiling (without lifting the chin) or being suspended from the ceiling by a string.

6) Tai chi has been promoted for improved health, memory, concentration, digestion, balance and flexibility. It may also aid in improving conditions such as anxiety, depression, and age-related declines in mental function. Studies have found that people who practice Tai chi are not as fearful of activity and are more confident when moving about. Tai chi includes movements that strengthen the legs. The exercises also provide an opportunity to explore where your center of gravity is, thereby exploring your balance. With practice you learn how to move your center of gravity. This can help you to become more aware of when you are getting unsteady and when you are not. As you begin to get things mapped out in your head, you gain more confidence, become more precise in your reactions, and more conscious of when you may be putting yourself at risk for a fall.

Tai chi Movements

Pressing Energy Down

Check your posture before you begin. Shoulders should be back and down and over the hips. Knees should remain slightly bent. Tuck in the chin and think about pushing the crown of the head up to the ceiling without lifting your chin. The abdominal muscles are lightly pulled in, but not so much that it restricts your breathing.

Stand with the feet shoulder to hip width apart and knees slightly bent. Arms are down by your side with the palms facing forward. Raise your arms to shoulder height with the palms facing the ceiling. Turn the hands so the palms face the floor, and slightly bend the elbows and wrists. Bring the arms back down to your side. Repeat eight to twelve times. Practice deep belly breathing. Allow your breath to be slow and deep throughout the movement. Repeat eight to twelve times. Allow your breath to be slow and deep throughout the movement, but do not try to coordinate your breath with the movement.

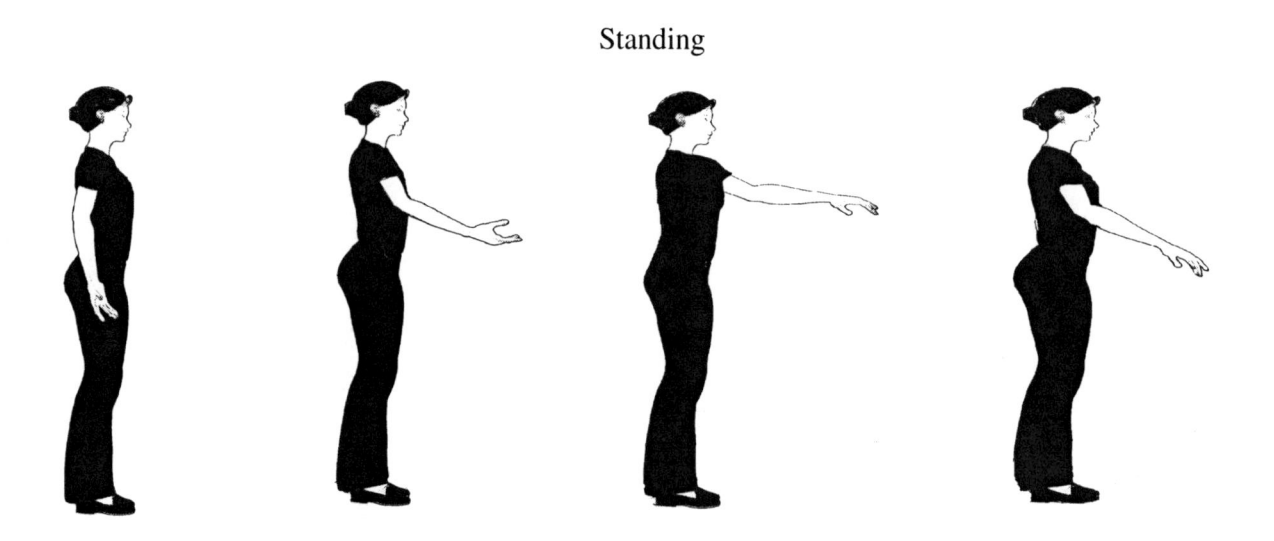

Standing

Seated

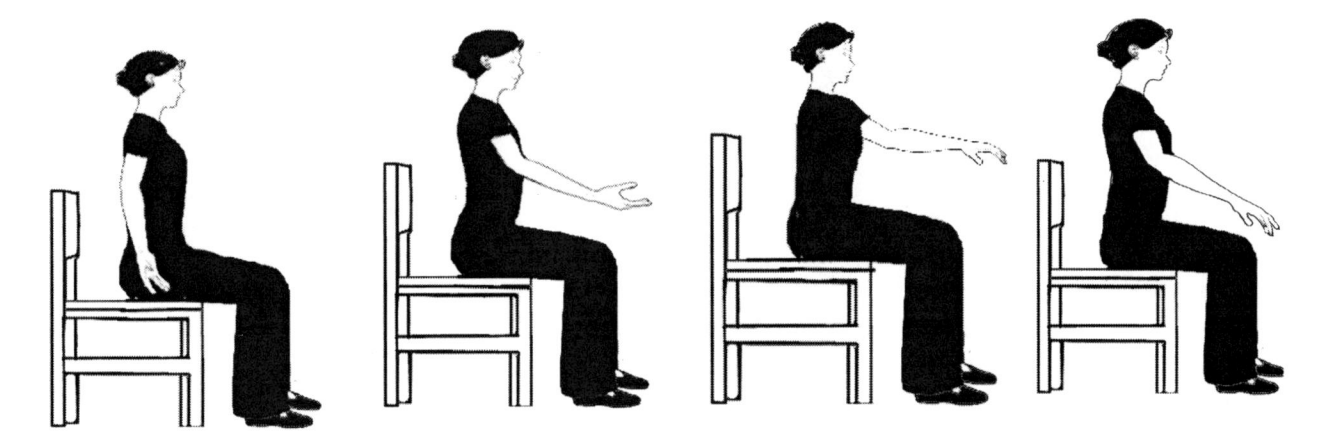

Checklist
- ✓ Stand or sit up straight
- ✓ Keep the shoulders down away from the ears
- ✓ Keep the natural curve in the low back
- ✓ Keep the knees, elbows and wrists soft and slightly bent
- ✓ Use diaphragmatic breathing through the nose as much as possible
- ✓ To further challenge your balance, you can try closing the eyes during this exercise
- ✓ Do not exercise to the point of strain or discomfort

Spreading the Eagle's Wings

Check your posture before you begin. Shoulders should be back and down and over the hips. Knees should remain slightly bent. Tuck in the chin and think about pushing the crown of the head up to the ceiling without lifting your chin. The abdominal muscles are lightly pulled in, but not so much that it restricts your breathing.

Stand with your feet shoulder to hip width apart and knees slightly bent. Arms are in front of the body in a circle. Lift your arms in front of the body (as if you were hugging a tree) and then into a circle overhead. With the arms overhead, turn the palms to face away from each other. Slightly bend the elbows and wrists. Bring the arms back down to your side. Repeat eight to twelve times. Allow your breath to be slow and deep throughout the movement, but do not try to coordinate your breath with the movement.

Standing

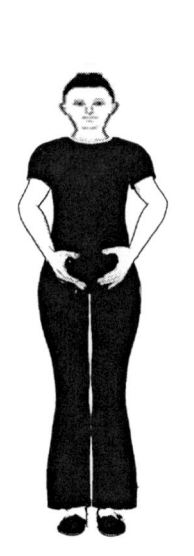

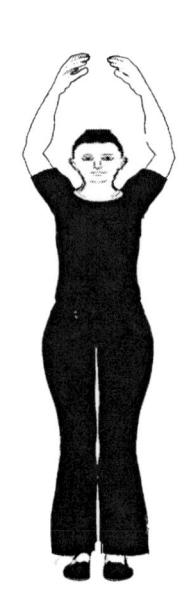

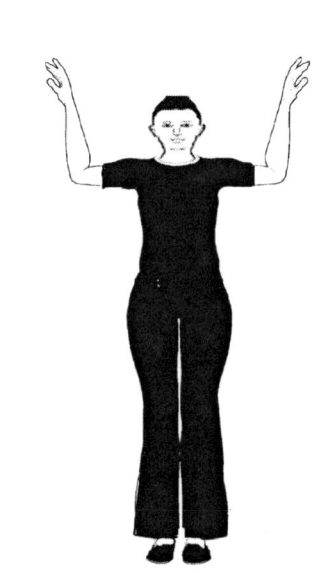

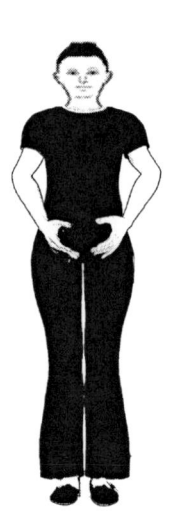

Seated

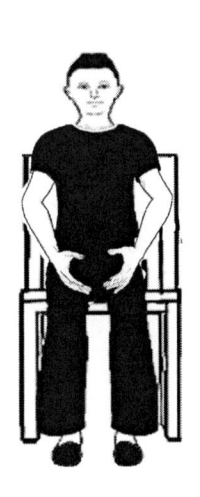

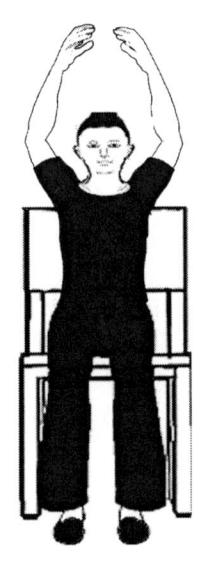

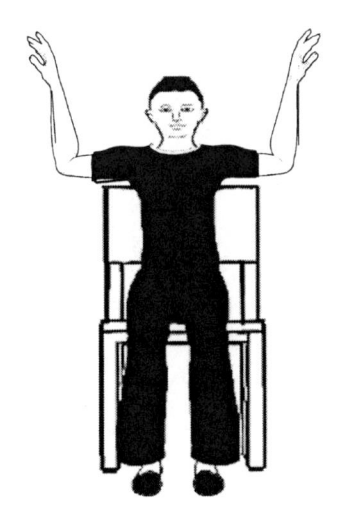

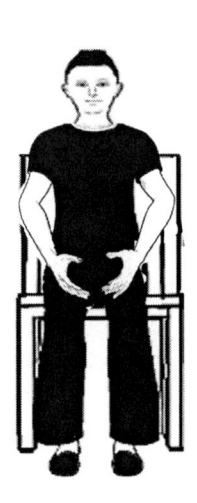

Checklist
- ✓ Stand or sit up straight
- ✓ Keep the shoulders down away from the ears
- ✓ Keep the natural curve in the low back
- ✓ Keep the knees, elbows and wrists soft and slightly bent
- ✓ Use diaphragmatic breathing through the nose as much as possible
- ✓ To further challenge your balance, you can try closing the eyes during this exercise
- ✓ Do not exercise to the point of strain or discomfort

Gathering Energy

Check your posture before you begin. Shoulders should be back and down and over the hips. Knees should remain slightly bent. Tuck in the chin and think about pushing the crown of the head up to the ceiling without lifting your chin. The abdominal muscles are lightly pulled in, but not so much that it restricts your breathing.

Stand with feet shoulder to hip width apart and knees slightly bent. Arms are by your sides with the arms and shoulders rotated out and the palms facing away from you. Raise the arms shoulder height with the palms facing the ceiling. Bring the palms towards each other at forehead height, forming a triangle with the arms. With the palms facing down, press the hands towards the floor. Finish by bringing the arms back to your side. Repeat eight to twelve times. Allow your breath to be slow and deep throughout the movement, but do not try to coordinate your breath with the movement.

Standing

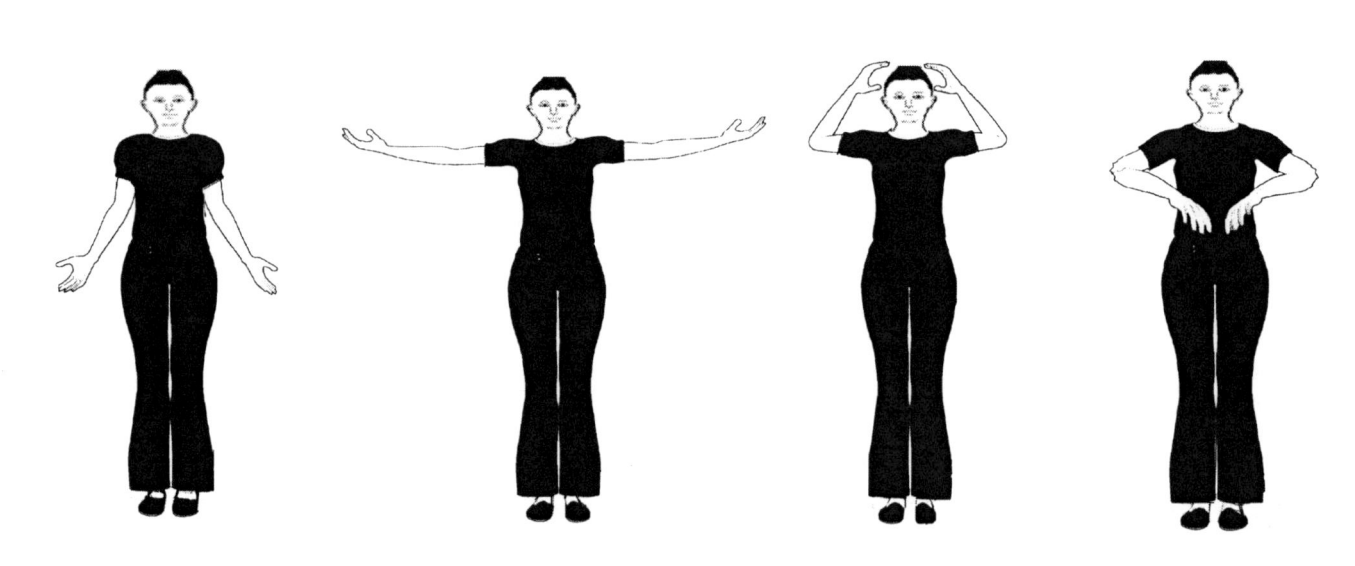

Seated

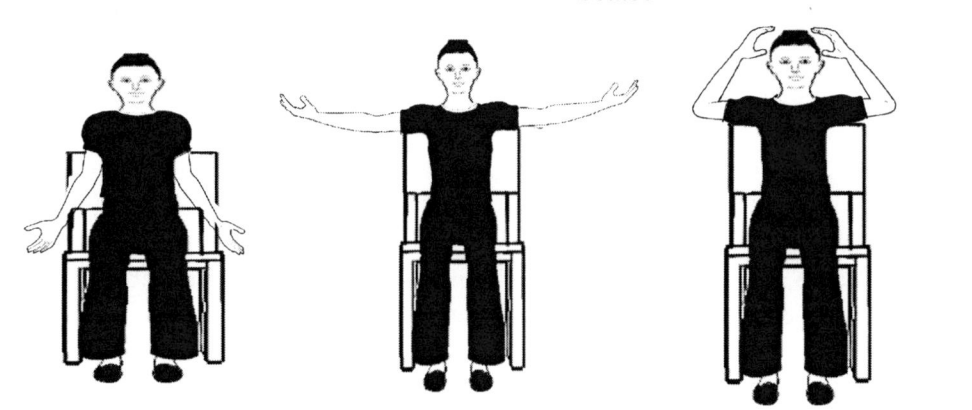

Checklist
✓ Stand or sit up straight
✓ Keep the shoulders down away from the ears
✓ Keep the natural curve in the low back
✓ Keep the knees, elbows and wrists soft and slightly bent
✓ Use diaphragmatic breathing through the nose as much as possible
✓ To further challenge your balance, you can try closing the eyes during this exercise
✓ Do not exercise to the point of strain or discomfort

Waist Twists

Check your posture before you begin. Shoulders should be back and down and over the hips. Knees should remain slightly bent. Tuck in the chin and think about pushing the crown of the head up to the ceiling without lifting your chin. The abdominal muscles are lightly pulled in, but not so much that it restricts your breathing.

If you have any back sensitivities use caution with this movement. Check with your health care provider if you have any concerns about the appropriateness of twisting motions.

Stand with the feet shoulder to hip width apart and knees slightly bent. Turning at the waist, press the right arm forward and your left arm straight behind you. Flex the hands and press through the palms to fully stretch the wrists and shoulders. Look back at your left hand. *Do not turn at the knees. The knees point straight ahead as you turn at the waist.* Come back to the center. Repeat on the left. Repeat 8-12 times to each side. Allow your breath to be slow and deep throughout the movement, but do not try to coordinate your breath with the movement.

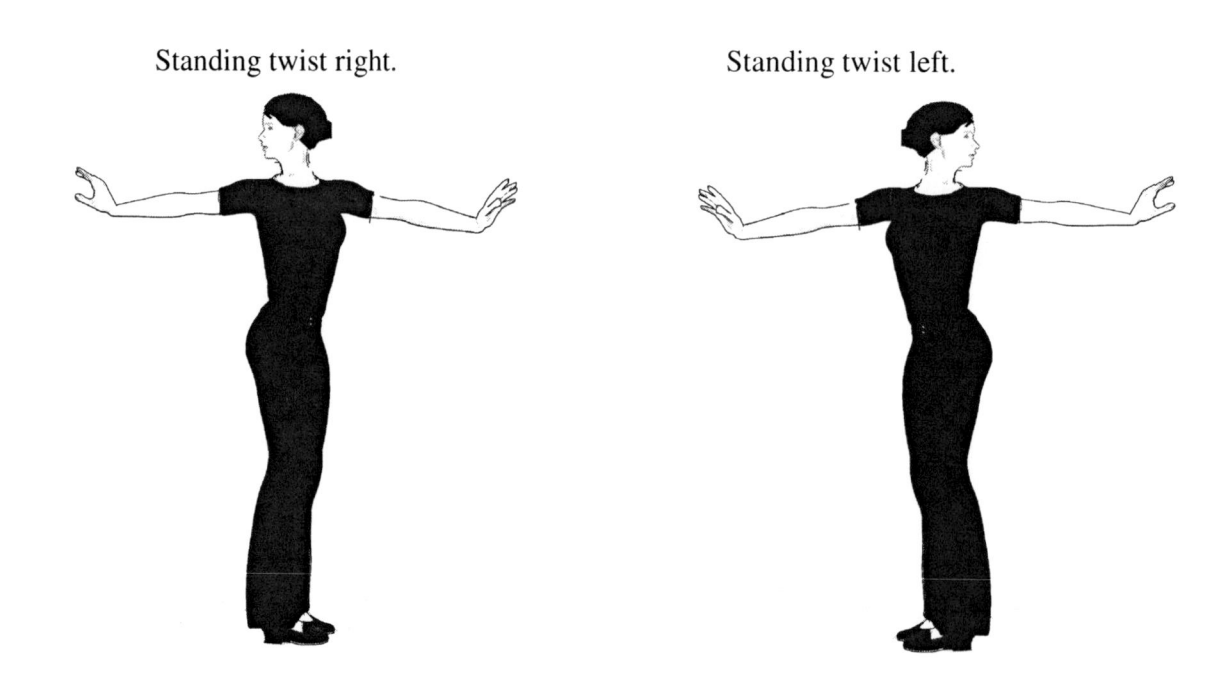

Standing twist right.

Standing twist left.

Seated twist right.   Seated twist left.

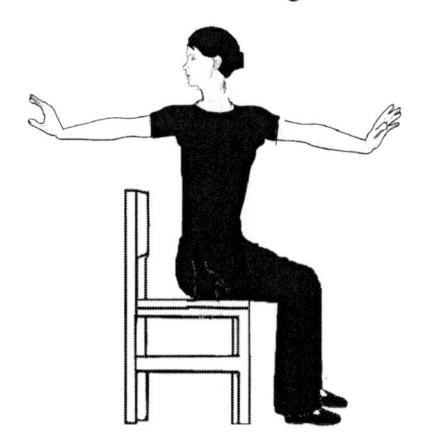

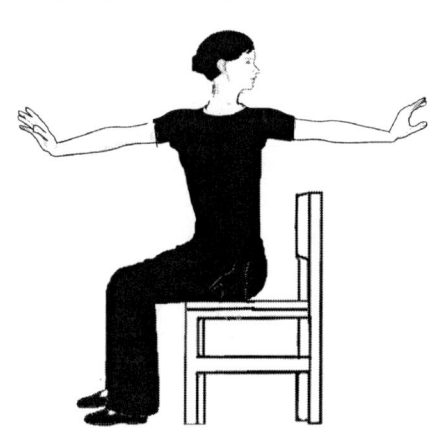

Checklist
- ✓ Stand or sit up straight
- ✓ Keep the shoulders down away from the ears
- ✓ Keep the natural curve in the low back
- ✓ Keep the knees, elbows and wrists soft and slightly bent
- ✓ Twist at the waist and keep the knees pointed forward
- ✓ Use diaphragmatic breathing through the nose as much as possible
- ✓ To further challenge your balance, you can try closing the eyes during this exercise
- ✓ Do not exercise to the point of strain or discomfort

Side Bends

Check your posture before you begin. Shoulders should be back and down and over the hips. Knees should remain slightly bent. Tuck in the chin and think about pushing the crown of the head up to the ceiling without lifting your chin. The abdominal muscles are lightly pulled in, but not so much that it restricts your breathing.

   Stand with the feet hip width apart and knees slightly bent. Bend to the right and press the right palm down towards the knee and the left palm up to the ceiling. Flex the hands and press through the palms to fully stretch the wrists and shoulders. Look up at your top hand. *Do not twist as you bend the shoulders and the hips stay facing straight ahead. Pretend you are between two panes of glass and can only bend to the side.* Come back to the center. Repeat to the left. Repeat 8-12 times to each side. Allow your breath to be slow and deep throughout the movement, but do not try to coordinate your breath with the movement.

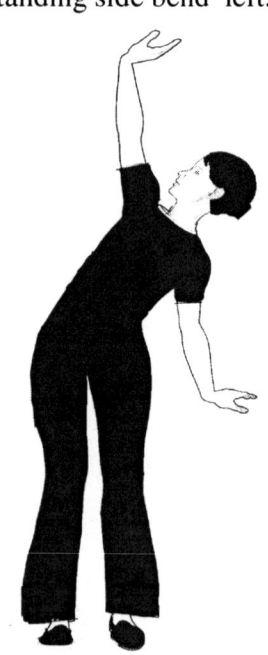

Standing side bend right.

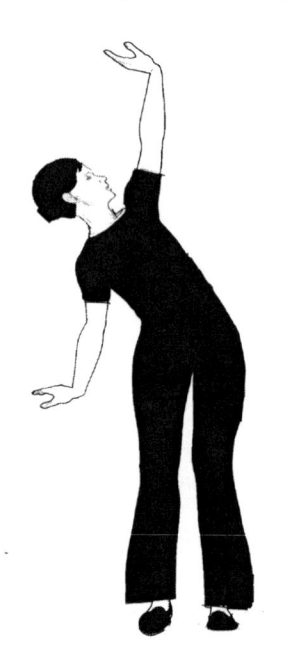

Standing side bend left.

Seated side bend right.   Seated side bend left.

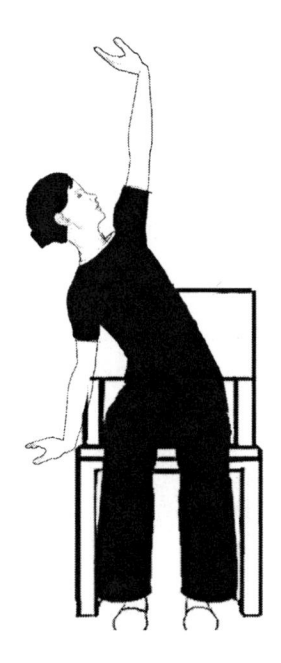

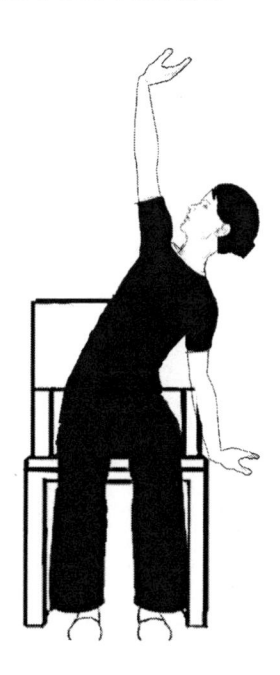

Checklist
- ✓ Stand or sit up straight
- ✓ Keep the shoulders down away from the ears
- ✓ Keep the natural curve in the low back
- ✓ Keep the knees, elbows and wrists soft and slightly bent
- ✓ Just bend to the side without twisting
- ✓ Use diaphragmatic breathing through the nose as much as possible
- ✓ To further challenge your balance, you can try closing the eyes during this exercise
- ✓ Do not exercise to the point of strain or discomfort

Tai chi Walk

This is meant to be a traveling movement and is only shown standing. If your balance is challenged you can do this exercise in a hallway using your hands against the wall for support or walk along next to a counter top.

Check your posture before you begin. Shoulders should be back and down and over the hips. Knees should remain slightly bent. Tuck in the chin and think about pushing the crown of the head up to the ceiling without lifting your chin. The abdominal muscles are lightly pulled in, but not so much that it restricts your breathing.

Bend the right knee lifting the right foot off of the floor. Bend the elbows and lift the lower arms up with the palms facing the ceiling. Place the right heel on the floor as the palms turn and push forward. Lower the right toes and lunge forward as the arms straighten out to the front. Step the left foot up to the right foot as the arms lower to your side.

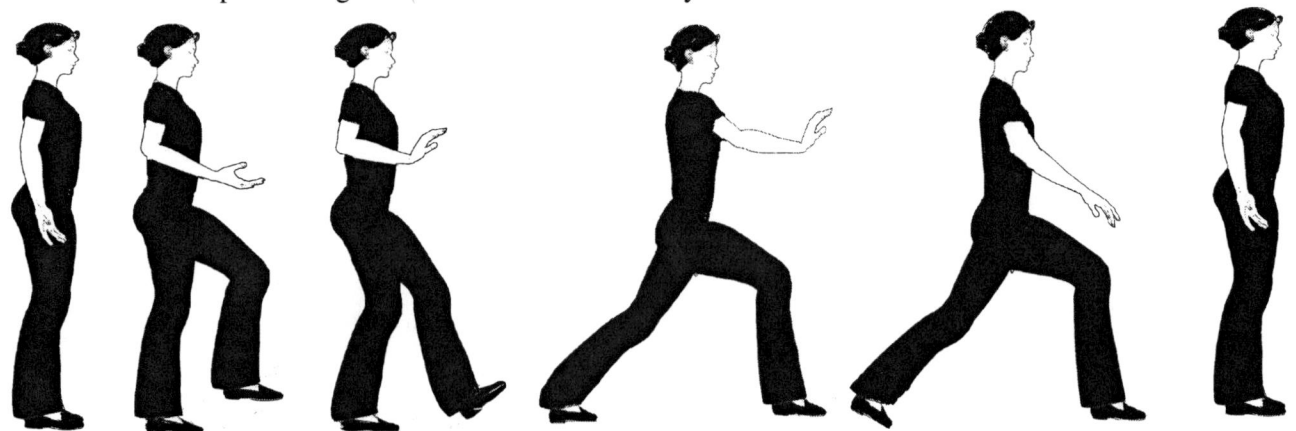

Repeat with the left foot.
Bend the left knee lifting the left foot off of the floor. Bend the elbows so the palms face the ceiling. Place the left heel on the floor as the palms turn and push forward. Lower the left toes and lunge forward as the arms straighten out to the front. Step the right foot up to the left foot as the arms lower to your side. Repeat eight to twelve times. Allow your breath to be slow and deep throughout the movement, but do not try to coordinate your breath with the movement.

Checklist
✓ Stand up straight
✓ Keep the shoulders down away from the ears
✓ Keep the natural curve in the low back
✓ Keep the knees, elbows and wrists soft and slightly bent
✓ Take smaller steps or hold onto a counter top or wall if balance is difficult
✓ Use diaphragmatic breathing through the nose as much as possible
✓ Do not exercise to the point of strain or discomfort

Chasing Clouds

This movement is a traveling movement to help improve balance and is only shown standing. If you find your balance is challenged you can do the leg movements while holding onto a counter or table.

Check your posture before you begin. Shoulders should be back and down and over the hips. Knees should remain slightly bent. Tuck in the chin and think about pushing the crown of the head up to the ceiling without lifting your chin. The abdominal muscles are lightly pulled in, but not so much that it restricts your breathing.

Hands are at your right side with the left hand on top like you are holding a small ball. Look to the right. Bend your left knee and pick up your left foot as high as you can keeping your balance. Step out to the left. Land in a squat position with *equal weight on both feet*. Turn the hands so that the right hand is on top. Keep the legs still as you carry the pretend ball to the center. Next, step the right foot to the left as you bring the hands and the pretend ball to your left side. Look to your left. Then bring the hands back to the right. Change so the left hand is on top again, and you are looking right. Repeat three more times to the left. Reverse the directions, traveling four times right. Take slow deep breaths but do not try to coordinate your breath with the movement.

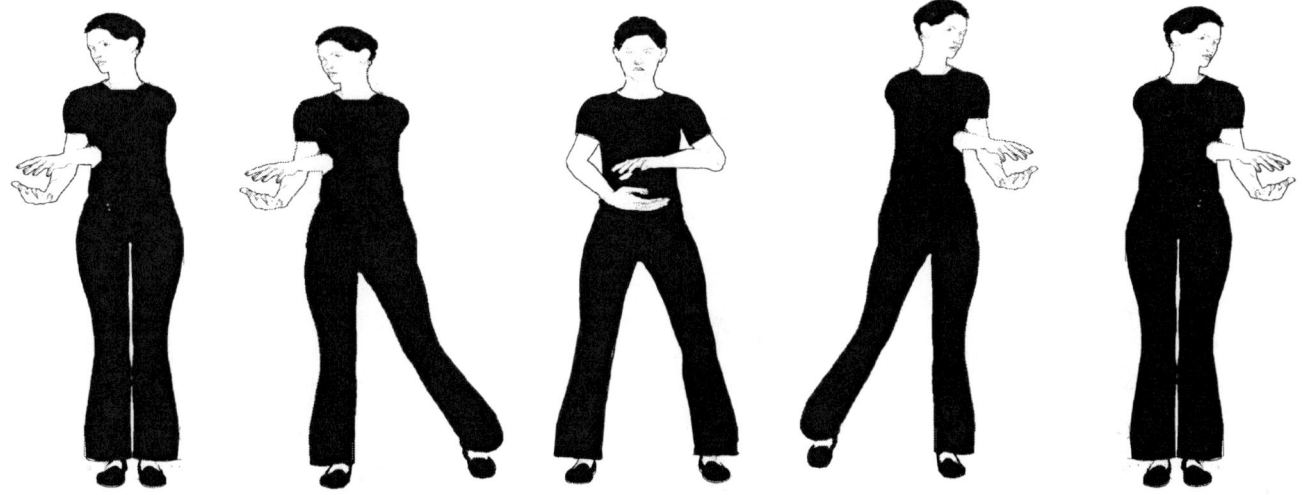

Checklist
- ✓ Stand up straight
- ✓ Keep the shoulders down away from the ears
- ✓ Keep the natural curve in the low back
- ✓ Keep the knees, elbows and wrists soft and slightly bent
- ✓ Take smaller steps if balance is difficult or hold onto a counter top
- ✓ Use diaphragmatic breathing through the nose as much as possible
- ✓ Do not exercise to the point of strain or discomfort

Tandem Walking

Another exercise that is helpful for balance is called Tandem Walking. This exercise is not a traditional tai chi movement but it is very good for improving balance. It involves slowly walking forward and backward with the feet tight together. If you find this challenging you can do this exercise walking down a hallway with your hands on the walks or walk along with one hand on a counter top.

Stand up straight with the left foot in front of the right. Next, step the right foot in front of the left with the heel flexed and the heel of the front foot touching the toe of the back foot. Then repeat putting the left foot forward so the left heel and right toes are touching. To get the most from this exercise make sure the heel and toes touch and do not separate the feet. Take a few steps forward. Take slow deep breaths but do not try to coordinate your breath with the movement.

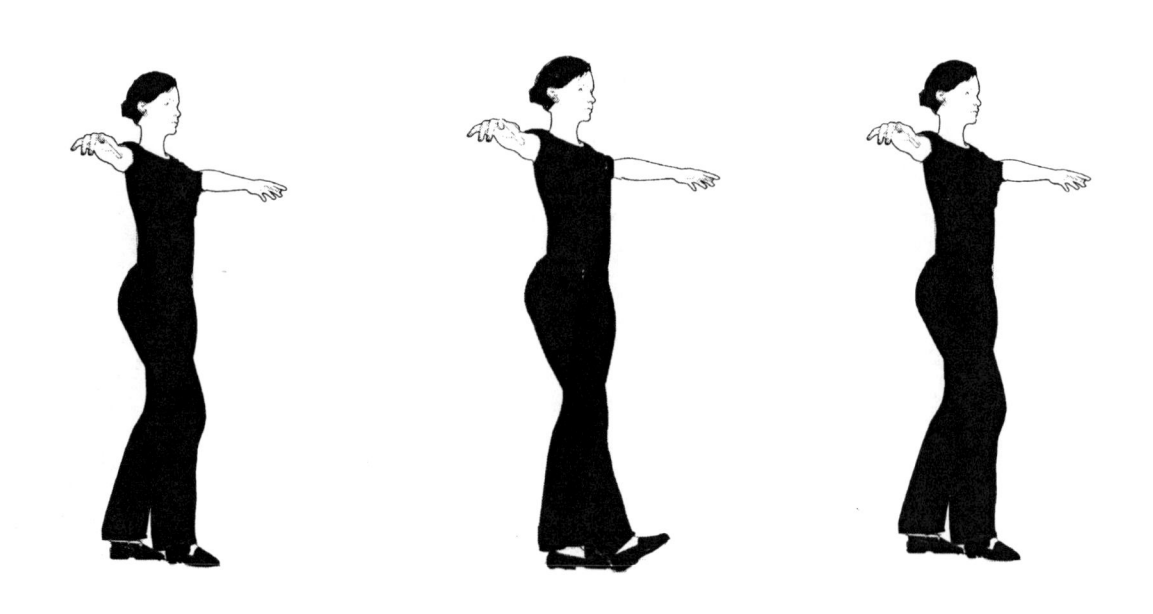

Then repeat going backwards. Place the right foot behind the left with the right toes touching the left heel. Then reach the left foot back touching the left toe and right heel. Take a few steps backwards. Take slow deep breaths but do not try to coordinate your breath with the movement.

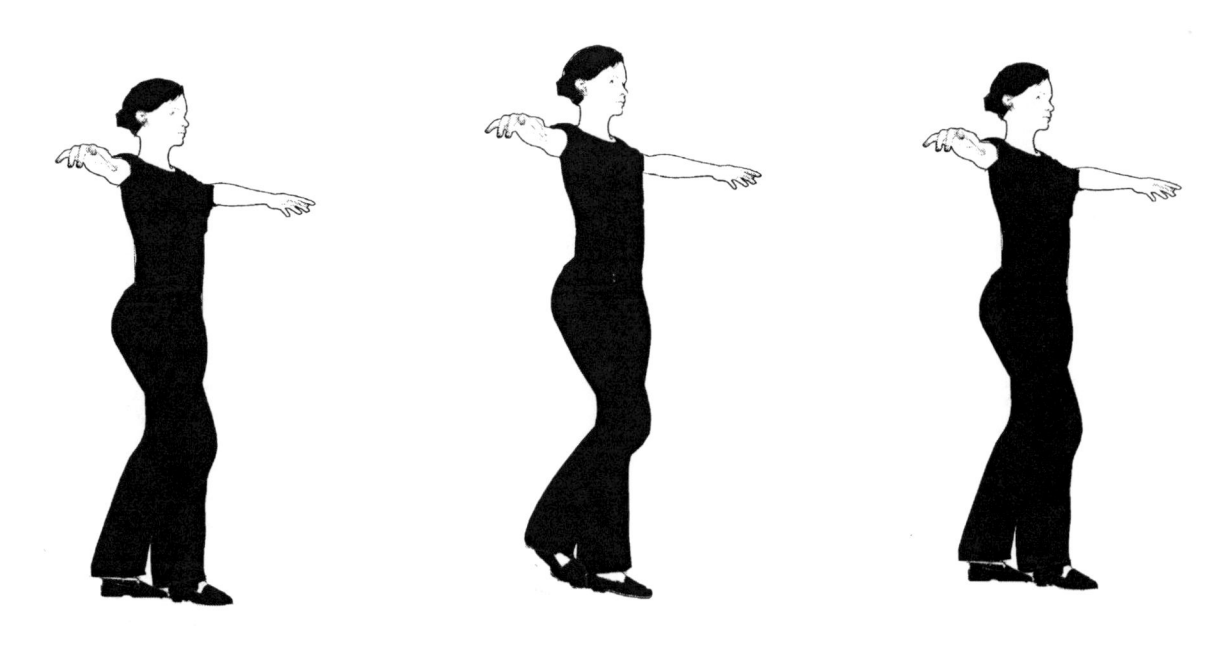

Checklist
✓ Stand up straight
✓ Keep the shoulders down away from the ears
✓ Keep the natural curve in the low back
✓ Go slowly and work on maintaining balance the entire time
✓ Use diaphragmatic breathing through the nose as much as possible
✓ Do not exercise to the point of strain or discomfort

Summary

A yoga and tai chi practice can be a great addition to an aerobic and strength training routine. Regular stretching is essential to help those with Parkinson's disease maintain range of motion and the body awareness gained through yoga and tai chi will help to reduce the risk of falls.

For best results you can vary your routine by performing aerobics and strength training exercises three times a week and practice yoga or tai chi postures on two or three alternate days. This will give you a well rounded program to help manage all of your symptoms. However, if you are experiencing significant trouble speaking, eating or projecting your voice you may want to practice the facial and voice projection exercises for ten to fifteen minutes every day.

Another component of yoga is learning to manage stress. The next chapter will address how stress can affect your body and Parkinson's symptoms. It also outlines several techniques you can try to help reduce tension.

> "My wife and I love to go out to dinner but having PD made it difficult to sit up a table for any length of time. The flexibility exercises in this book helped to improve my posture and range of motion so that I could once again sit at a table and have dinner with my wife"
>
> - C.F. Massachusetts

Chapter 6
Relaxation Techniques and Stress Management.

"Courage doesn't always roar. Sometimes courage is the little voice at the end of the day that says I'll try again tomorrow."

-- Mary Anne Radmacher

Stress is not a disease but rather a normal part of everyone's life. Stress is any event that an organism must adapt to, and it does not necessarily have a negative or positive correlation. Stress results from situations that require one to change and/or adjust behaviorally and such changes can be positive or negative. Examples of stress include the body responding to the pressures of gravity, physiological adaptations to an exercise regimen, or changes to one's way of life. Stress can include feelings of mental or emotional strain, suspense, anxiety, fear, worry, tension, excitement, or a general feeling of uneasiness or dread in response to a real or imagined threat. Any sort of change can make you feel stressed, even good change. It's not just the change or event itself that matters, but how you react to it. Therefore the word stress does not always need to be associated with a negative event. What may be stressful is different for each person. For example, although one person may not feel stressed about retiring from work, another person may. Getting married is a joyous event. It is also stressful for many. Having to adjust to an illness or financial changes can be stressful. In life, we have to constantly adjust to change. Exposure to stress becomes a issue when the stressor is perceived as something to which one can not adapt to, control, or when an individual believes that he or she is unable to cope with the situation.

Effects of Stress on the Body

Stress is caused by the body's natural instinct to defend itself. In the case of emergencies such as getting out of the way of a speeding car this instinct is good, but it can cause physical symptoms if it goes on for too long, such as in response to life's daily challenges and changes. Stress evokes the fight-or-flight response. The fight-or-flight response is characterized by increased metabolism, heart rate, breathing, and blood pressure all of which prepare us to run or to fight. In order for this to occur, the various systems of the body must signal and communicate with one another. The body accomplishes this communication through the use of messenger molecules that send and receive signals to activate both voluntary and involuntary actions. Some of the systems of the body involved include the nervous system, the neuropeptide system, the immune system, and the endocrine system.

The Nervous System
This system is comprised of the central nervous system (CNS) and the peripheral nervous system. The peripheral system connects the CNS to sensory receptors and motor neurons

allowing the CNS to communicate with the muscles and glands. The peripheral nervous system is further divided into the autonomic nervous system which includes the sympathetic nervous system and the parasympathetic nervous system.

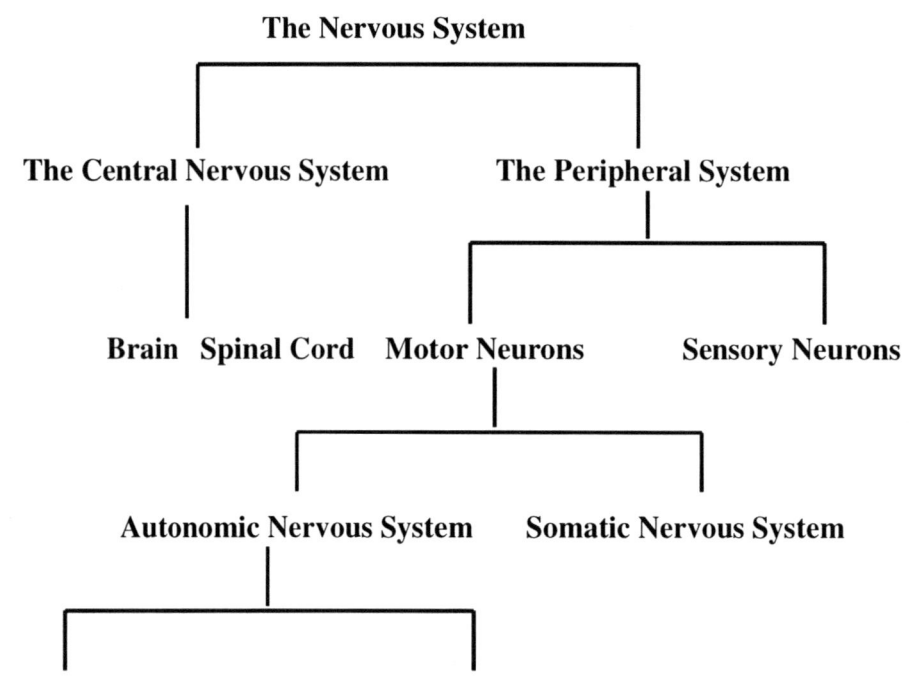

```
                        The Nervous System
                    ┌──────────────┴──────────────┐
        The Central Nervous System          The Peripheral System
                    │                     ┌──────────┴──────────┐
            Brain  Spinal Cord       Motor Neurons        Sensory Neurons
                                  ┌──────────┴──────────┐
                        Autonomic Nervous System    Somatic Nervous System
                        ┌──────────┴──────────┐
            Sympathetic Nervous System    Parasympathetic Nervous System
```

Understanding the Stress Response

Constant exposure to even mild stress over a prolonged period of time may have a detrimental effect on the body. In cases where there is a threat to our survival or physical well being the stress response is activated as needed, but then it is deactivated when the threat has passed. However, problems occur when the stress response is not deactivated. The stress response can become a constant occurrence in our daily life such as during an argument, being stuck in traffic, experiencing financial difficulties, or when facing a chronic illness. While these situations may not be life threatening, whenever the body-mind senses that we are worried or "stressed" the fight or flight response is stimulated. If we constantly feel the pressures of such situations during daily life, then our body-mind is in a constant state of arousal.

The stress response occurs when an individual is exposed to a perceived danger. Then, in less then a second, the sympathetic nervous system (SNS) is signaled to release catecholamines such as epinephrine (adrenaline) and norepinephrine (noradrenaline), that enhances rapid activation of our reflex response system.

These chemicals cause an increase in heart rate, muscle tension, and blood pressure. Blood flow is diverted from the internal organs and skin, and sent to the brain and muscles. Our rate of breathing increases, our pupils dilate, and perspiration increases. The hypothalamus, interpreting the above reactions, relays information to the molecule corticotrophin-releasing hormone (CRH) as well as to other hormones. These hormones then signal the pituitary gland to release adrenocorticotrophin (ACTH) as well as other hormones in order to evoke additional adaptive responses. These adaptive responses include the release of cortisol which aids in mobilizing energy, increasing cardiovascular and cardiopulmonary activity, sharpening cognitive abilities to increase performance, and decreasing the activity of the immune and digestive systems.

After you've fought, fled or otherwise escaped your stressful situation, the parasympathetic nervous system is signaled to reverse the above process bringing the body back to a "resting" state as the levels of cortisol and adrenaline in your bloodstream decline. As a result, your heart rate and blood pressure return to normal and your digestion and metabolism resume their regular pace.

The Autonomic Nervous System and the Fight Or Flight Response

Parasympathetic System – Calms the body down	Sympathetic System – activates the body to run or fight
Constricts Pupils	Dilates pupil
Stimulates salivation	Inhibits salivation
Slows heartbeat	Accelerates heartbeat
Slows breathing	Accelerates breathing
Stimulates digestion	Inhibits digestion
Inhibits hormones	Activates secretion of hormones
Contracts bladder	Relaxes bladder
Relaxes rectum	Contracts rectum

Stress Response Triggers

First, it is essential to understand that the brain does not always know the difference between a real and imagined threat, for example; you are watching a frightening movie. Even though you may be sitting comfortably in your living room and reason tells you that you are not actually in danger, your body still responds. When you see frightening images the brain interprets these as a danger or threat to the well being of the body, and in turn activates the fight or flight response. Your heart beat increases, your breathing quickens and becomes more shallow, your palms may become sweaty, and you may even physically jump or become startled. While at a much lower level this same set of reactions can occur due to a constant stream of negative thoughts or during periods of constant worry. These thoughts and worries are signals to the brain that something is wrong or that there is a threat to your well being, causing the body to respond. This reaction can occur even if the thoughts you are having are merely anticipations about what might happen. Frequently our worries are about events that have not actually happened.

Stress and Your Health

As explained above, the human body is designed to experience stress and to react to it. Stress can be positive, keeping us alert and ready to avoid danger. Stress becomes negative when a person faces continual challenges without relief or relaxation between challenges. When stressful situations pile up one after another, your body has no chance to recover. As a result, one may tend to become overworked as stress related tension builds. Stress that continues without relief can lead to physical symptoms including headaches, upset stomach, elevated blood pressure, chest pain, and problems sleeping. The long-term activation of the stress-response system can disrupt almost all your body's processes, increasing your risk of obesity, insomnia, digestive complaints, heart disease, and depression. Stress can also bring on or worsen certain symptoms or diseases. Stress is linked to some of the leading causes of death such as heart disease, cancer, lung ailments, accidents and cirrhosis of the liver. Chronic stress can wear down the body's natural defenses and cause health problems or make problems worse if you don't learn ways to deal with it.

Stress can effect such systems of the body as:

Digestive System
It's common to have a stomachache or diarrhea when you're stressed. This happens because stress hormones slow the release of stomach acid and the emptying of the stomach. The same hormones also stimulate the colon, which speeds the passage of its contents. Chronic stress can also lead to continuously high levels of cortisol. This hormone can increase appetite and cause weight gain.

Immune System.
Chronic stress tends to decrease the activity of your immune system, making you more susceptible to colds and other infections. Normally, your immune system responds to infection by releasing several substances that cause inflammation. In response, the adrenal glands produce cortisol, which switches off the immune and inflammatory responses once the infection is cleared. However, prolonged stress keeps your cortisol levels continuously elevated, so your immune system remains suppressed. In some cases, stress can have the opposite effect, making your immune system overactive. The result is an increased risk of autoimmune diseases where your immune system attacks your body's own cells.

Nervous System

If your fight-or-flight response never shuts off, stress hormones produce persistent feelings of anxiety, helplessness and impending doom. Oversensitivity to stress has been linked with severe depression, possibly because depressed people have a harder time adapting to the negative effects of cortisol. The byproducts of cortisol act as sedatives, which contribute to the overall feeling of depression. Excessive amounts of cortisol can cause sleep disturbances, a lessening of the sex drive and loss of appetite.

Cardiovascular System

High levels of cortisol can also raise your heart rate and increase your blood pressure and blood lipid (cholesterol and triglyceride) levels. These are risk factors for both heart attacks and strokes. Cortisol levels also appear to play a role in the accumulation of abdominal fat, which gives some people an "apple" shape. People with apple body shapes have a higher risk of heart disease and diabetes than do people with "pear" body shapes, where weight is more concentrated in the hips.

Other Systems

Stress may worsen such skin conditions as psoriasis, eczema, hives and acne, and it can be a trigger for asthma attacks.

Signs and Symptoms of Stress

Physical	*Behavioral*	*Emotional*
Headaches	Restlessness	Crying
Indigestion	Being overly critical of others	Nervousness
Stomach aches	Grinding one's teeth at night	Anxiety
Sweaty palms	Inability to get things done or make decisions	Boredom (there's no meaning to anything)
Hypertension (high blood pressure)	Easily upset	Edginess (a readiness to explode)
Dizziness or a general feeling of "being out of it"	Excessive anger and hostility	Feeling powerless to change things
Tension in the back, neck, face, and shoulders	Lack of creativity	An overwhelming sense of pressure
Heart rate/pulse irregularities	Problems with relationships	Loneliness
Insomnia		Depression
Tiredness		Constant worry
Trembling/shaking		Loss of sense of humor
Constipation or diarrhea		
Shortness of breath		

Stress and Parkinson's Disease

Current estimates by the National Parkinson's Foundation indicate that nearly half of all Parkinson's patients are anxious and depressed. Stress management is essential in the effective management of Parkinson's disease because all symptoms of Parkinson's disease (tremors, stiffness, and slow movements) can get worse under stress. The right amount of rest along with a regular program of stress management is a very important part of controlling the symptoms of Parkinson's disease. There is some suggestion that stressful life events can possibly accelerate the progression of disease in some patients.

Techniques to Manage and Reduce Your Stress

The following steps can help you to manage the effects of stress.

1. Learn to recognize when you're feeling stressed and become conscious of your reaction to the stress.
2. Choose a way to deal with your stress. Identify stressful events that you can change, eliminate or reduce exposure to. To the best of your ability prepare for events you know may be stressful (a job interview or doctor's appointment). If you can not avoid the situation, you can choose to change how you react to stress. Try to look at change as a positive challenge, not a threat.
3. Step back from the conflict or worry and shift your outlook. Many times, simply choosing to look at situations in a more positive way can reduce the amount of stress in your life.
4. Don't worry about things you can't control (the weather or another's actions). Teach yourself to control your physical reactions to stress.
5. Build up your emotional ability to deal with stress.
6. Ask for help from friends, family or professionals. Take a break, talk to someone close and get a different perspective on your troubles. Work to resolve conflicts with other people. On your own, you may have limited success trying to change the habitual patterns of thought and behavior that trigger your stress response. Psychiatrists, psychologists, and licensed clinical social workers are trained to help you break free of these patterns.
7. The most important step you can take is to seek help as soon as you feel less able to cope. Taking action early will enable you to understand and deal with the many challenges of Parkinson's disease.
8. Set realistic goals at home and at work.
9. Exercise on a regular basis. Exercise increases your physical capacity to deal with stress.
10. Eat well-balanced meals and get enough sleep. Get away from your daily stresses by participating in group sports, social events, and hobbies.
11. Remember, it is not your fault that you have Parkinson's disease. There is *no guilt* attached to having Parkinson's disease. You must believe this - consciously and subconsciously!

12. Take control. Exercise, join a support group, look outside yourself, help others. Everyone else in the Parkinson's community is in this with you. Find out as much as you can about the illness. Talk to your friends and family about it. Do not isolate them. They will want to be involved in helping you.
13. Learn to meditate or practice relaxation techniques
14. Lastly, EVERYDAY do something you enjoy.

Stress management requires continuous practice as you go through life and deal with change which often comes unexpectedly. Even if you take everyday frustrations in stride, your stress response can still surge up when you find yourself dealing with something big, such as illness, job loss, or bereavement. The remainder of this chapter will cover meditation and relaxation techniques you can use to manage stress.

Using Meditation and Relaxation Techniques

Meditation and relaxation techniques are forms of focused concentration that work by introducing calm, peaceful images in the mind, creating a "mental escape." Meditation techniques provide a powerful psychological strategy that enhances a person's coping skills. Many people dealing with stress feel loss of control, fear, panic, anxiety, helplessness, and uncertainty. In contrast practicing meditation and relaxation techniques can help you to overcome stress, anger, pain, depression, insomnia, and other problems associated with illnesses and medical/surgical procedures. Stress and depression can worsen the symptoms of Parkinson's disease. Meditation and relaxation techniques help you to remain calm. In addition to reducing stress and depression, meditation and relaxation techniques can dramatically decrease pain and the need for pain medication, decrease side effects and complications of medical procedures, shorten hospital stays and reduce recovery time, enhance sleep, strengthen the immune system, enhance the ability to heal, and increase self-confidence and self-control.

There are many types of meditation or relaxation techniques. All aim for the same outcome they simply utilize different techniques. Experiment with the different techniques in order to find one that works well for you. You may also find that some techniques work best in certain circumstances.

Basic Meditation or Relaxation Technique

When practicing this basic technique the physiological and psychological reactions that occur in the body are the exact opposite of those which happen during the activation of the fight or flight response. By regularly eliciting this calmer state, you may be able to counteract the detrimental effects of constant stress. When the fight or flight response is activated several reactions occur. These include an increase in heart rate, blood pressure, rate of respiration, muscular tension, and blood flow being directed away from the process of digestion and instead directed towards the muscles and brain. When the basic meditation exercise is practiced the exact opposite can occur. There may be a reduction in heart rate, rate of respiration, muscular tension, and an overall decrease in the body's metabolism.

    The goal of the basic meditation exercise is to allow the mind to shift away from the constant stream of thoughts and worries and instead focus solely on the movement of the breath. This helps to slow down the activity and chatter in the mind, which in turn will send signals to the body-mind that you are relaxed and there is nothing to worry about. As the body-mind receives these calming signals, the brain will signal the body to calm the nervous system and reverse the effects of the fight or flight syndrome. You may also find that after meditating you may be less likely to rush around and more inclined to remain in the peaceful state you achieved during your relaxation session. The following steps outline a general basic meditation practice.

1) Find a quiet place where you will not be disturbed for about fifteen to twenty minutes. Turn off phones and remove as many distractions as possible.

2) Find a comfortable position. This can be sitting in a chair with the back straight but not rigid and feet flat on the floor, or sitting cross-legged on the floor. If you find sitting cross-legged on the floor uncomfortable on your knees or back, you can sit on a cushion or pillow in order to raise your hips a bit higher then your knees. This will help to both take pressure off of the knees and maintain a straight back. You can also lie down for this exercise, as long as you do not fall asleep. Remember mediation is about developing a skill to use when stressed and falling sleep is not always an option, so work to stay awake during meditation and learn to focus the mind away from stressful thoughts.

3) Close the eyes and begin to focus on your breath.
Inhale through the nose and allow your abdominal area to rise, as if you were filling this area with air. Exhale through the nose and allow the stomach to fall as the air leaves this area. Sometimes it is easier to start with the exhalation and just once, contract the abdominal muscles and push the air out. Then allow the stomach to relax and rise with the inhalation. It is normal for this style of breathing to feel backwards or awkward at first but with practice it will become easier.

4) For the next twenty minutes remain focused on your breath. To keep the mind focused allow yourself to be aware of the abdomen as it rises and falls, or allow your attention to remain on the sensation of the air as it enters and exits the nose. If these sensations are difficult to focus on, the breath can be counted by silently saying one on the inhale and two on the exhale. If the mind does wander, which it will, simply without judgment bring your attention back to the breath. When the twenty minutes is up, allow yourself time and do not get up too quickly. Take a few minutes to feel the results of your meditation.

    When first attempting this exercise you may need to bring your attention back quite often. However, keeping your attention on the breath and away from other thoughts will become easier with practice. You can time yourself for the twenty minutes, however, avoid using a loud alarm as you do not want to startle the body out of meditation. An alarm which can be programmed to come on with soft music could be used. You can also choose some soft music that lasts for as long as yo want to meditate. It is not recommended to continually open the eyes and look at the time as this disrupts the process of concentrated meditation. Remember to keep a passive attitude. Meditation is a skill and like any new skill, takes practice. Remember to not get concerned about doing the exercise correctly and be careful about expecting any particular results. The object is to simply take time out of the day to give the body-mind a break from everyday thoughts and worries.

For all of the techniques presented in this book the breathing is taught in and out of the nose, since this is physiologically more relaxing for the body. However if you are experiencing respiratory or sinus issues and find this difficult, you can breathe in through the nose and out through the mouth with pursed lips. You may find that with practice, breathing strictly through the nose will become easier.

Autogenic Training (AT)
This technique trains the body to become quiet and relaxed by utilizing self-suggestions. These self-suggestions attempt to change the thoughts present in the mind, by suggesting to the brain that certain events are occurring. These events can include a slower heartbeat, increased blood flow, and less muscle tension. Since it is possible that negative thoughts can result in decreased efficiency of the systems in the body, advocates of AT suggest that we can utilize positive thoughts to enhance the efficiency of the systems of the body.

If you find that the following suggestions do not apply to your situation, please feel free to substitute any other "suggestions." You may wish to record these instructions onto a tape until you are more familiar with the process.

1) Find a comfortable position that you can remain in for about twenty minutes where you will not be disturbed. Begin to focus on your breath and allow your body to relax. Slowly and silently count down from four to one. When you reach the number one you will be completely relaxed.

2) Concentrate on your right arm. Slowly and silently say to yourself six times, my right arm is very heavy.
Concentrate on your left arm. Slowly and silently say to yourself six times, my left arm is very heavy.
Concentrate on both arms. Slowly and silently say to yourself six times, my arms are very heavy. Turn your attention away from your arms, and silently say to yourself just once, I am very quiet, and I enjoy feeling relaxed for a while.

3) Concentrate on your right leg. Slowly and silently say to yourself six times, my right leg is very heavy.
Concentrate on your left leg. Slowly and silently say to yourself six times my left leg is very heavy.
Concentrate on both legs. Slowly and silently say to yourself six times my legs are very heavy.
Turn your attention away from your legs, and silently say to yourself just once, I am very quiet, and I enjoy feeling relaxed for a while.

4) Concentrate on the beating of your heart. Slowly and silently say to yourself six times, my heartbeat is calm and strong.
Turn your attention away from your heartbeat, and silently say to yourself just once, I am very quiet and I enjoy feeling relaxed for a while.

5) Concentrate on the rhythm of your breathing. Slowly and silently say to yourself six times, my breathing is slow and deep.
Turn your attention away from your breath and silently say to yourself just once, I am very quiet and I enjoy feeling relaxed for a while.

6) Concentrate on your stomach. Slowly and silently say to yourself six times, warmth is radiating throughout my stomach and throughout my body.
Turn your attention away from your stomach and silently say to yourself just once, I am very quiet and I enjoy feeling relaxed, for a while.

7) Concentrate on your forehead. Slowly and silently say to yourself six times, my forehead is cool.
Turn your attention away from your forehead and silently say to yourself just once, I am very quiet and I enjoy feeling relaxed, for a while.

8) Bring your attention back to your breath.

9) Slowly and silently count down from four to one. By the time you reach the number one, you will be alert and awake, yet relaxed. Begin to circle the wrists and ankles, gently stretching and moving the body. When you are ready, slowly open the eyes. Take a few minutes to feel the effects of your meditation.

Guided Imagery

Where Autogenic Training utilizes self-suggestion, guided imagery relies on images to suggest physiological changes to the brain to create harmony between the mind and body. Guided imagery or visualization is a process by which you create calm, peaceful images in your mind in order to help elicit a state of relaxation or manage symptoms. Guided imagery, much like the basic meditation exercise, aims to present the brain with different stimuli to focus on, allowing for a break from everyday thoughts and worries. Imagery is often used to stimulate changes in bodily functions that are usually considered inaccessible to conscious influence. Imagery can be effective since the brain will respond to mentally created images much in the same way it responds to actually seeing images. A common example of how this works is to try the following exercise.

First try to imagine a lemon... Use all of your senses... Smell the lemon and get a sense of its texture... Next, recall what a lemon tastes like... Now imagine cutting open the lemon and squirting some of the lemon juice into your mouth... Imagine swishing the lemon juice around in your mouth and then swallowing it.

In this exercise even though tasting the lemon was only in your imagination you may have noticed changes in your body. You might have begun to salivate and you might have even puckered at the thought of the taste. In this example your body responded to the thought as though the event actually took place. Constant worry is another example of the effects of imagery. As you worry about events that may or may not happen, your body may respond by tensing muscles and arousing the nervous system in anticipation of a challenge.

Imagery can also provide a way to communicate conscious intentions or requests to your unconscious mind. When using guided imagery the participant might visualize a scene such as a beach, meadow, or other such place which can elicit feelings of relaxation and peace. In this example when imagining such a scene, the brain receives signals that it is all right to relax since there is no threat present. Imagery may also be used when dealing with a particular disease such as cancer. In this case the patient may use imagery to visualize the body healing itself from the disease by "seeing" or imagining their immune system eliminating the cancerous cells. Imagery, like many of the complementary techniques available can be used in conjunction with medical treatment. For someone who is taking medication for an illness, imagery could be used to visualize the treatment working. For those with Parkinson's disease this could mean visualizing the body having enough dopamine present and the body moving smoothly. As with most all forms of meditation, the practice of guided imagery or visualization can help to interrupt the flow of constant thoughts and worries, and thereby allow the body and mind to rest, conserve energy, and build energy reserves.

Using guided imagery (or other types of meditation) to manage stress and symptoms can provide a sense of hope and encourage feelings of control over one's situation. However, as with any form of meditation, a passive attitude is essential. While it is important to make the images as real as possible, it is just as important to not focus on results or particular outcomes. When an end result or outcome is the focus, anxiety and tension can result which are counterproductive to stress and symptom management.

When first practicing guided imagery it may seem difficult to actually "see" the images. It is important to know that with practice, visualizing images will become easier. It is important to not become frustrated or tense if visualization exercises do not come easily. Sometimes it may be easier to "sense" the image versus struggling to "see" the image. For example if trying to visualize a healing light, instead of "seeing" the light you may choose to just "sense" that it is there, by focusing on a sensation of warmth or heat, a tingling sensation, or just simply knowing that it is there.

In order to practice guided imagery you can try a simple exercise. Notice a basic object around your home. Make it something simple without a lot of design. Observe the object for a few minutes and really notice its detail. Then, close your eyes and try to recall the object in your mind's eye. Try this with various objects keeping it simple at first, and then work up to more detailed objects.

There are many different versions of guided imagery exercises, however the example below is a commonly used technique. It will be easier to either record the instructions on a tape or have someone read them to you so you can remain focused on the process versus continually having to stop and look at the directions. As with the basic meditation exercise, find a way to time yourself so you are not startled out of the meditation. You will need approximately twenty minutes for this exercise.

1) Begin by practicing the basic meditation technique for approximately five to ten minutes. The time does not need to be exact, but it should be long enough for you to feel a shift in the state of tension and relaxation of your body. The following is the script to use for the imagery section. Where I have included "….." signals a time to give yourself a few moments in-between the next instruction.

2) Begin to imagine yourself walking on a private beach on a perfect summer day………Take some time to look around and use all of your senses to explore the area………Hear the waves as they come up gently on the shore………. Feel the warm sun on your skin and the sand underneath your feet…………Smell the salt air……….. notice how being here makes you feel……………Find a place where you can sit or lie down either on the shore, in the water, or anywhere else that looks inviting to you…………..Begin to become aware of the light and warmth from the sun…………. As you relax here allow this warmth and light to permeate your skin and be absorbed into the body…..Allow yourself to imagine this light and warmth to have healing properties…………. If there are any areas of tightness, tension, or disease present in the body-mind allow these things to be dissolved by the warmth and light……………. Take some time here to relax and heal the body…… (*allow ten to fifteen minutes here for this experience . If*

you make a tape or someone is guiding you through this experience periodically have reminders to bring your attention back to the meditation and away from distracting thoughts).

Begin to bring your attention back to the breath…… Feel the abdomen rise as you inhale and the abdomen fall as you exhale……..Allow yourself to slowly and gently become a little more awake and a little more alert with each breath………….. become aware of the pressures against your body from the floor or chair………..Then when you are ready slowly open the eyes.

3) Allow yourself to come out of the meditation slowly and take some time to feel the effects of the exercise.

4) Remember to maintain a passive attitude. Visualizing images can be difficult at first, however, it will become easier with practice. If you find visualizing the above difficult, you can try to focus on sensation instead. In this example, you would allow yourself to feel the sensation of being at a relaxed spot, and focus more on the sensation of the warmth of the sun entering your body versus focusing on actually visualizing the light.

Mindfulness Meditation

This form of meditation, which has its roots in Buddhism, is focused on learning to become fully present in the moment and to be accepting of whatever is occurring in the present moment. Unlike the three other forms of meditation presented, this form of meditation aims to help the participant change their response to stimuli rather then alter their physiology. The goal is for the meditator to be fully aware of the stimuli around them, (such as noise or other people), yet learn to not react to the stimuli. This process is also referred to as learning to become a dispassionate watcher or a witness. During this process the participant aims to become aware of the mind's constant stream of thoughts and to it's constant judgment and reaction to inner and outer experiences. This technique aims to teach one how to not get caught up in these thoughts by allowing oneself to step back from the thoughts. This form of meditation is based on a fundamental Buddhist belief - that the origin of much of our suffering comes from a constant need to grasp onto things and the attempt to change what is.

An example of this would be meditating while experiencing pain. In the basic meditation exercise, the participant tries to interrupt the pain signals, and the typical anxiety laden thoughts that accompany them, by shifting the mind's attention onto awareness of the breath, since interrupting the flow of thoughts can often aid in reducing symptoms. Autogenic Training would utilize self-suggestions such as the area which is painful, is becoming more relaxed and is therefore more comfortable. In the case of guided imagery the participant might try mentally visualizing the pain as a red ball which then turns into a softer color and becomes smaller and smaller until the ball disappears. With these types of meditation the aim is to interrupt the stream of thoughts which are occurring in the mind, but also suggest to the brain that the pain no longer exists.

However, when using mindfulness meditation, the participant would not attempt any of the above. Rather the meditator would acknowledge the pain but attempt to not react to it with thoughts of anger, depression or frustration. Approaching the sensation of pain in this way gives the mind an alternate way of seeing discomfort. Instead of becoming agitated by the sensation the meditator would relate to the experience or sensation of pain simply as an event that is happening in the present, but would refrain from allowing the mind to wander to negative thoughts about the sensation. In other words the meditator would not allow the mind to become distracted with thoughts which attempt to predict what the pain may or may not do in the future, or how the pain effects their life. This process attempts to run interference so that thoughts, emotions and/or memories do not integrate the experience of pain with the activation of the fight or flight response. This form of meditation can help the participant to learn to lessen the times the body is activated when exposed to stress.

Below is a sample of a typical mindfulness meditation exercise. As with the other forms of meditation, find a way to time yourself for twenty minutes so you will not be startled out of the exercise.

1) Begin by practicing the basic meditation technique for approximately five to ten minutes. The time does not need to be exact, but it should be long enough for you to feel a shift in the state of tension and relaxation of your body.

2) When your mind has quieted down, try shifting your awareness to the process of thinking and take your attention off of the breath. Attempt to be a dispassionate observer as you simply "watch" the thoughts which come into your mind. Try to perceive the thoughts simply as events in your mind. Try to not allow yourself to become caught up in the thoughts, just notice that they are there. Notice their content and the rate at which they change. Notice that each particular thought does not last very long, but rather individual thoughts come and go, and sometimes the same thought will keep coming back. If you notice sensations of discomfort, allow yourself to become aware of the sensations, yet choose to not react to them. Notice if the sensations change with time. Again try to practice being the observer of an event. Notice if by simply observing the sensation you can allow yourself to become detached from the sensation. (However if you are experiencing significant discomfort do not force yourself to continue with this exercise).

3) To end the meditation bring your awareness back to your breathing for a few minutes. Come out of the meditation slowly and allow yourself a few minutes to experience the effects of this exercise.

4) Remember to maintain a passive attitude. Try to avoid getting caught up in how well you performed the meditation or becoming attached to any particular results.

This form of meditation can be challenging at first. You may find it difficult to stay with this exercise for a full twenty minutes. If this occurs, start by practicing for just a few minutes at a time and slowly build up to a fifteen to twenty minute practice.

Summary

This book has covered many techniques and forms of movement, which can help in managing the symptoms and challenges faced by those with Parkinson's disease. In addition there are many other opinions, approaches, and techniques not covered in this book. We encourage you to explore all of the options available and try many different approaches. With exploration you will find the approach that works best for your unique situation.

On the following pages are various workout logs, diaries, sample exercise routines and lists of helpful websites for more information. Use these resources as a guide to help you find the best program for your body. As you continue to experiment with different ideas and techniques you will eventually be able to work out a routine on your own. Always remember to listen to your own body to know if an exercise or technique is right for you. Exercise should always leave you feeling better then before, not worse. If you notice new symptoms or an increase in current symptoms after starting this or any other program, stop the exercise and check with your doctor or physical therapist about how best to proceed. Usually it is only a matter of making some minor adjustments to the routine you are doing in order for you to continue.

Appendix

The following pages provide sample routines, workout logs, and suggestions for using the information in this book and developing a regular exercise program. These are provided as a guide only to help you in getting started in developing your own routine. As you learn how different movements affect you, you can then work to develop your own routine. The following are general suggestions concerning the use of movement therapy for those with Parkinson's disease.

For the best results, you need to do some exercise everyday. You do not need to do all of the exercises in this book every day. It is best to alter your routine between a variety of exercises. Doing the same exact workout every time you exercise will cause the body to adapt to the routine and lessen the affect of the exercise. To keep the body responding to exercise it is important to periodically change your routine or change the amount or type of resistance you are using. The following list provides information on the exercises that are important to do everyday and exercises which are best if done two or three times per week

Things you should try to do everyday to manage your PD symptoms include:
1) Deep diaphragmatic breathing exercises. Try for ten to fifteen minutes of deep breathing each day. This helps to reduce stress and improves lung capacity and speech volume.
2) Stretching to bring the shoulders back and open the chest. This is important to help correct a forward rounded posture.
3) Balancing exercises to help prevent falls.
4) Facial exercises to counter any speech or swallowing issues..
Things you should do at least two to three times per week.
1) Aerobic or cardiovascular exercise. This can either be the aerobic exercises from chapter three or walking. During the week you can alternate the aerobic exercises with a brisk fifteen to thirty minute walk. You should walk at a pace that gets your heart rate up and you should feel slightly out of breath. Make sure you use correct walking form (pg. 27) using heel-toe walking and swing your arms (opposite arm to leg). An indicator of good cardiovascular health is being able to complete a fifteen-minute mile. This may be too fast of a pace, but gives you something to aim for.
2) Strengthening exercises for the arms, legs, and abdominal muscles.
3) A full body stretching routine.
Things you should do at least once per week.
1) Get down on the floor and practice getting back up (page 42) . Keep yourself in practice of getting up and down off of the floor. Then if you do fall, you will be limber enough to get up on your own without having to wait for assistance.

Sample Weekly Routine One

You do not need to do the exercises all at the same time, they can be done throughout the day. Remember, the following routines are *"the ideal"* involving some exercise every day. There may be times when you miss your workout or are not feeling up to exercise, or are only able to do part of it. Use your own judgment as to what is best for your body, and how much exercise is appropriate. Make a commitment to exercise as often as you realistically can and be gentle with your body when needed.

These routines take approximately one hour per day.

Monday
Warm-up exercises.
Aerobic exercises.
Strength training exercises.
Facial exercises.
Ten to fifteen minutes of deep breathing with or without a meditation technique.

Tuesday
Walk for fifteen to twenty minutes or to tolerance.
Yoga exercises.
Voice projection exercises.
Ten to fifteen minutes of deep breathing with or without a meditation technique.

Wednesday
Warm-up exercises.
Aerobic exercises.
Strength training exercises.
Facial exercises.
Ten to fifteen minutes of deep breathing with or without a meditation technique.

Thursday
Walk for fifteen to twenty minutes or to tolerance.
Tai Chi exercises.
Voice projection exercises.
Ten to fifteen minutes of deep breathing with or without a meditation technique.

Friday
Warm-up exercises.
Aerobic exercises.
Strength training exercises.
Facial exercises.
Ten to fifteen minutes of deep breathing with or without a meditation technique.

Saturday
Warm up exercises
Some type of aerobic exercise different from walking or the aerobic exercises in this book.
Examples include swimming, biking, water walking, or some sport you enjoy.
Voice projection exercises.
Ten to fifteen minutes of deep breathing with or without a meditation technique.

Sunday
Pick an activity you enjoy to get the body moving and challenge your balance.
Ten to fifteen minutes of deep breathing with or without a meditation technique.

Sample Weekly Routine Two

Monday
Warm-up exercises.
Aerobic exercises.
Upper body strength training exercises.
Facial exercises.
Ten to fifteen minutes of deep breathing with or without a meditation technique.

Tuesday
Walk for fifteen to twenty minutes or to tolerance.
Lower body strength training exercises.
Yoga exercises.
Voice projection exercises.
Ten to fifteen minutes of deep breathing with or without a meditation technique.

Wednesday
Warm-up exercises.
Aerobic exercises.
Upper body strength training exercises.
Facial exercises.
Ten to fifteen minutes of deep breathing with or without a meditation technique.

Thursday
Walk for fifteen to twenty minutes or to tolerance.
Lower body strength training exercises.
Tai Chi exercises.
Voice projection exercises.
Ten to fifteen minutes of deep breathing with or without a meditation technique.

Friday
Warm-up exercises.
Aerobic exercises.
Upper body strength training exercises.
Facial exercises.
Ten to fifteen minutes of deep breathing with or without a meditation technique.

Saturday
Warm up exercises
Some type of aerobic exercise different from walking or the aerobic exercises in this book.
Examples include swimming, biking, water walking, or some sport you enjoy.
Voice projection exercises.
Ten to fifteen minutes of deep breathing with or without a meditation technique.

Sunday
Pick an activity you enjoy to get the body moving and challenge your balance.
Ten to fifteen minutes of deep breathing with or without a meditation technique.

Warm Up Exercises Reference Sheet

    You can use the reference sheets and logs below to help you design your workout. Once you become familiar with the various exercises and the number of repetitions to do, you can use these reference sheets as a quick checklist to help you remember the movements. It is important to read the complete instructions to make sure you are performing the exercises correctly and to avoid injury to the joints. Remember most of the standing exercises can also be done holding on or seated in a chair if needed.

Half neck rolls/neck stretch pg. 52

Head rotation and stretch pg. 55

Chin tuck pg. 57

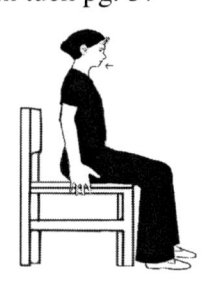

Shoulder rolls pg. 58

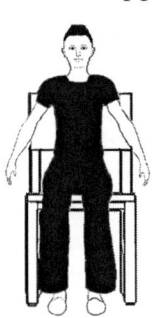

Spinal twist/stretch pg. 59

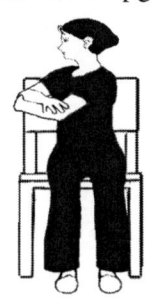

Cat stretch pg. 62

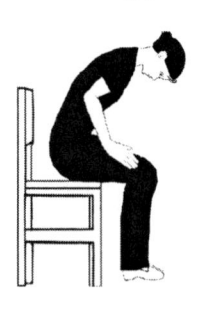

Chest opener pg. 63

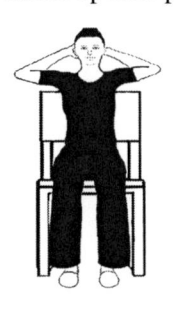

Toe lifts pg. 65

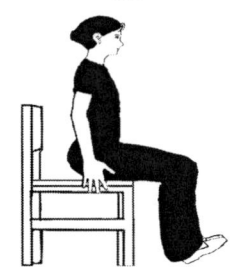

Heel lifts pg. 66

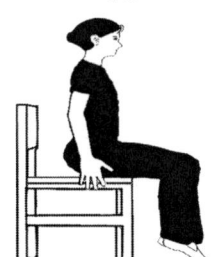

Side bend. 67

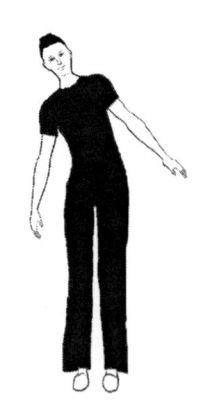

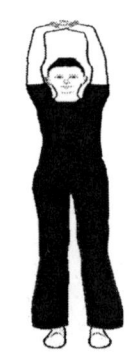

Side Stretch 69

Arm circles pg. 71

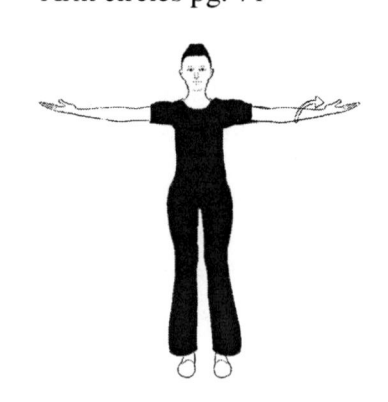

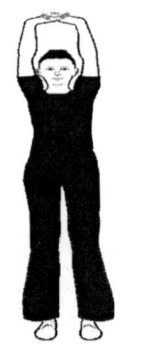

Squat pg. 72

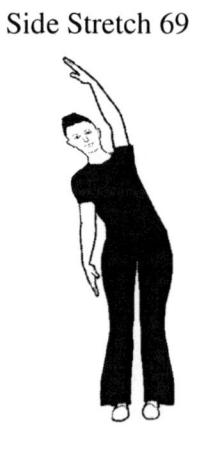

Overhead stretch pg. 74

Chest stretch pg. 75

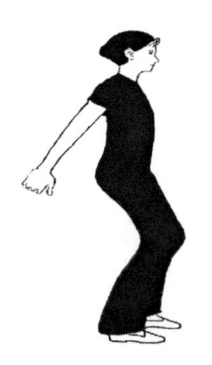

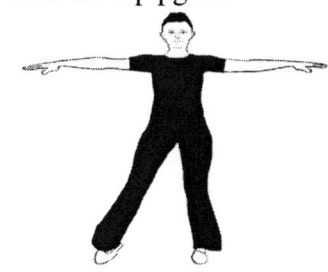

Aerobic Exercises Reference Sheet

Refer to Chapter three for complete instructions. These movements can also be done holding on or seated.

March in place pg. 85

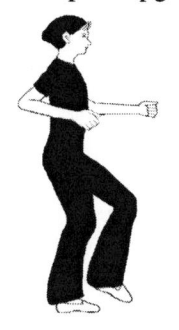

Straight leg kicks. pg. 86

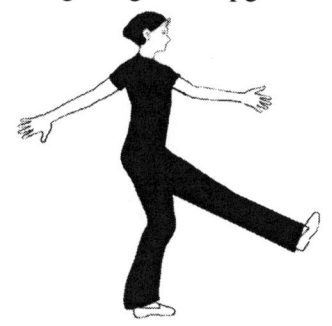

Step side to side pg. 87

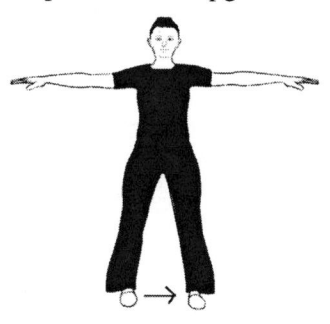

Knee lifts pg. 89

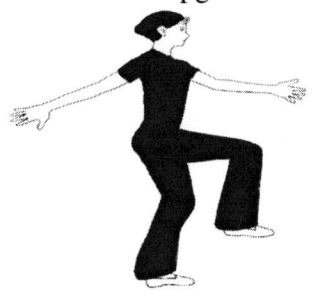

Heel curls pg. 90

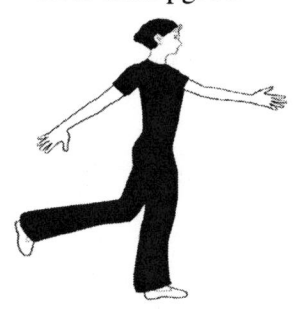

Side toe tap pg. 91

Heel taps pg. 93

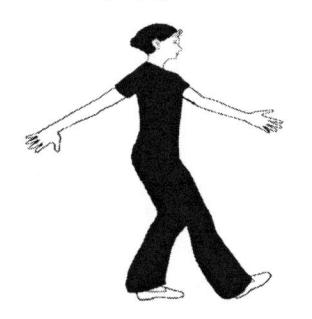

211

Workout log for aerobic exercises

Below is a sample log showing you how to fill it in.

Aerobic exercise log   Week of _01___/_05___/_04___

	Sun.	Mon.	Tues.	Wed.	Thurs.	Fri.	Sat.
March in place		1 min.		2 min.		1 min.	
Straight leg kick		1 min.		2 min.		1 min.	
Step side to side		1 min.		2 min.		1 min.	
Knee lifts		1 min.		2 min.		1 min.	
Heel curls back		1 min.		2 min.		1 min.	
Side toe taps		1 min.		2 min.		1 min.	
Heel taps		1 min.		2 min.		1 min.	
Walking			20 min.		15 min.		20 min.
Swimming	20 min.						

The following page has a blank sheet you can copy and use for your workouts.

Aerobic exercise log

Week of ____/____/____

	Sun.	Mon.	Tues.	Wed.	Thurs.	Fri.	Sat.
March in place							
Straight leg kick							
Step side to side							
Knee lifts							
Heel curls back							
Side toe taps							
Heel taps							
Walking							
Swimming							

Strength Training Exercises Reference Sheet

Refer to Chapter four for complete instructions. The standing movements can also be done seated.

Squats/Wall Slide pg. 99

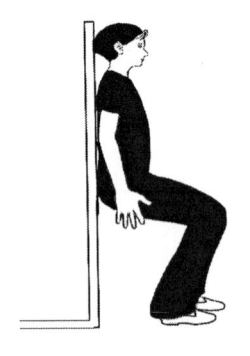

Leg extension. pg. 100

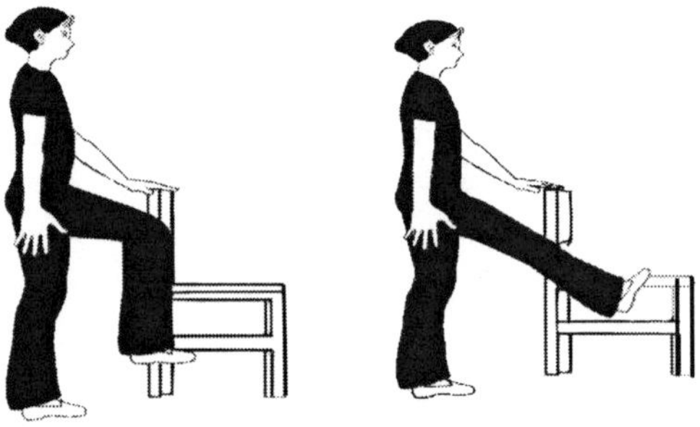

Side leg lift pg. 102

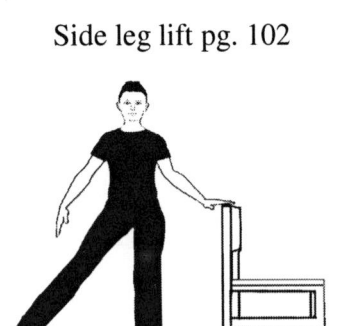

Leg lift back pg. 104

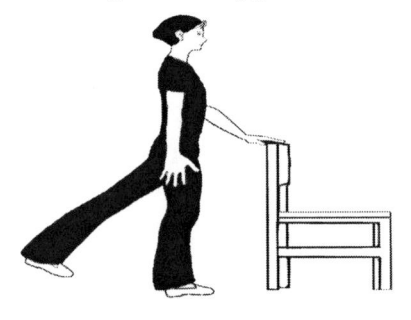

Leg crossover pg. 106

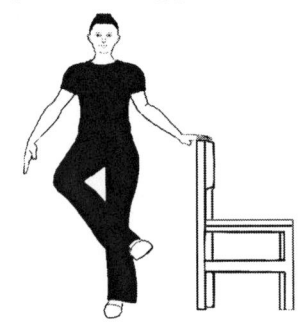

Heel raises pg. 108

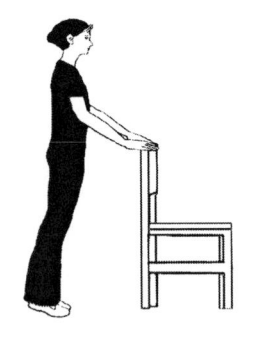

Toe Lifts pg. 110

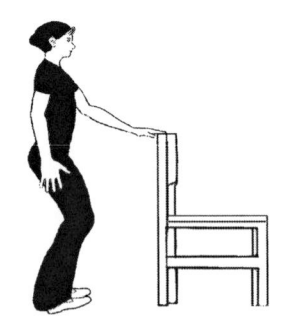

Wall pushups pg. 112

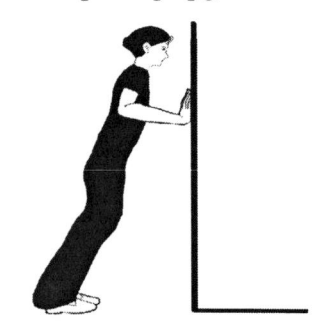

214

Chest fly pg. 113	Bent row pg. 114	Front lateral raise pg. 116
Military press pg. 117	Deltoid raise pg. 118	Biceps curl pg. 119
Triceps kickback pg. 120	Wrist curl pg. 121	Reverse wrist curl pg. 122

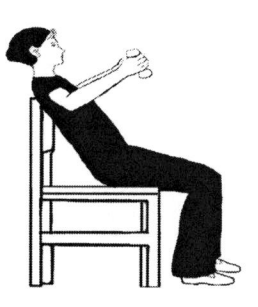

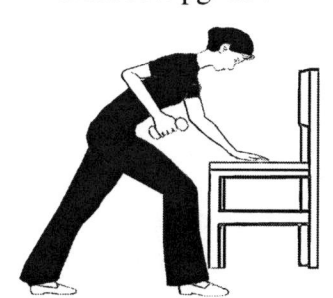

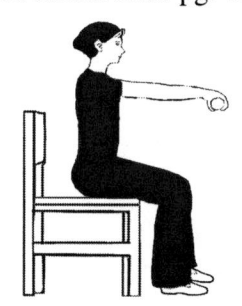

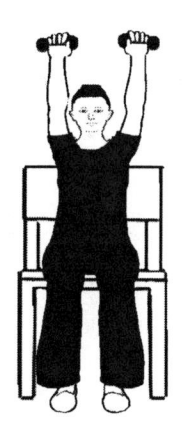

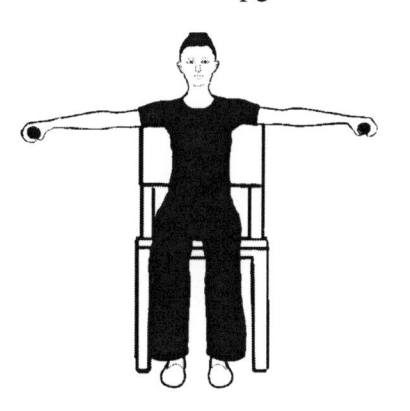

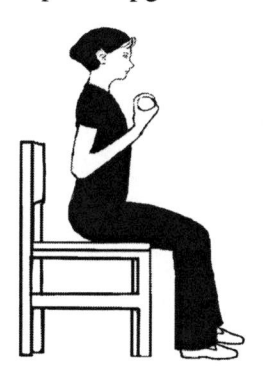

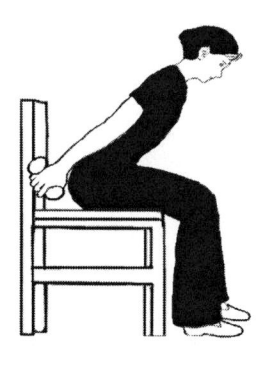

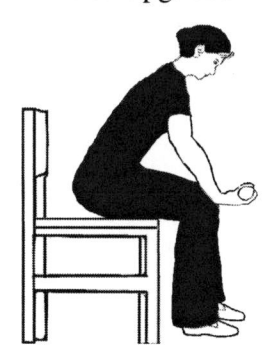

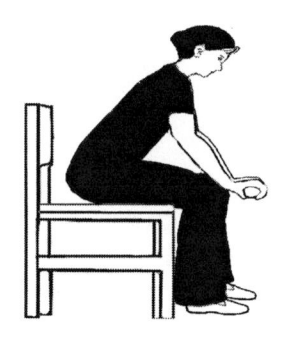

Abdominal lean backs pg. 123

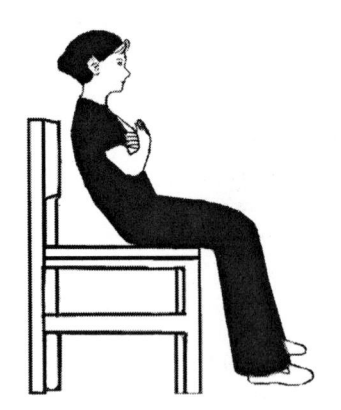

Bicycle pg. 124

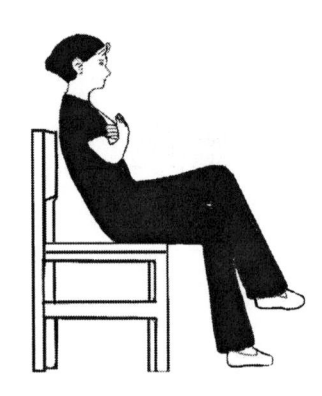

Side bends pg. 126

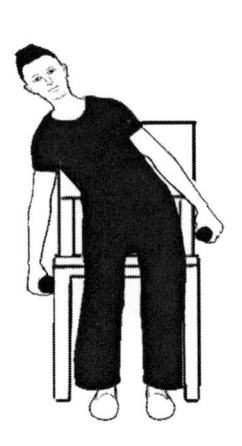

Workout log for Strength training exercises

Use this log to record the amount of weight you use and the number of repetitions you complete. Below is a sample log showing you how to fill it out.

*Strength training log   Week of __01__/__05__/__04_*

	Sun.	Mon.	Tues.	Wed.	Thurs.	Fri.	Sat.
Squat/Wall slide		10 reps 3 pounds		10 reps 3 pounds		10 reps 3 pounds	
Leg extension		10 reps		10 reps		10 reps	
Side leg lift		10 reps 3 pounds		10 reps 3 pounds		10 reps 3 pounds	
Leg lift back		10 reps 3 pounds		10 reps 3 pounds		10 reps 3 pounds	
Leg crossover		10 reps 3 pounds		10 reps 3 pounds		10 reps 3 pounds	
Heel raises		10 reps 3 pounds		10 reps 3 pounds		10 reps 3 pounds	
Toe Lifts		10 reps 3 pounds		10 reps 3 pounds		10 reps 3 pounds	
Wall Pushups		10 reps		10 reps		10 reps	
Chest fly		10 reps 3 pounds		10 reps 3 pounds		10 reps 3 pounds	
Bent row			10 reps 2 pounds		10 reps 2 pounds		10 reps 2 pounds
Front lateral raise			10 reps 2 pounds		10 reps 2 pounds		10 reps 2 pounds
Military press			10 reps 2 pounds		10 reps 2 pounds		10 reps 2 pounds
Deltoid raise			10 reps 2 pounds		10 reps 2 pounds		10 reps 2 pounds
Biceps curl			10 reps 2 pounds		10 reps 2 pounds		10 reps 2 pounds
Triceps kickback			10 reps 2 pounds		10 reps 2 pounds		10 reps 2 pounds
Wrist curls			10 reps 2 pounds		10 reps 2 pounds		10 reps 2 pounds
Reverse wrist curls			10 reps 2 pounds		10 reps 2 pounds		10 reps 2 pounds
Lean backs		12 reps		12 reps		12 reps	
Bicycle		10 reps		10 reps		10 reps	
Side bends		12 reps		12 reps		12 reps	

On the following page is a blank log you can make copies of to keep track of your progress.

Strength training log

Week of ____/____/____

	Sun.	Mon.	Tues.	Wed.	Thurs.	Fri.	Sat.
Squat/Wall slide							
Leg extension							
Side leg lift							
Leg lift back							
Leg crossover							
Heel raises							
Toe Lifts							
Wall Pushups							
Chest fly							
Bent row							
Front lateral raise							
Military press							
Deltoid raise							
Biceps curl							
Triceps kickback							
Wrist curls							
Reverse wrist curls							
Lean backs							
Bicycle							
Side bends							

Yoga Reference Sheet

Refer to Chapter five for complete instructions. The standing movements can also be done seated.

Mountain pose pg. 135

Forward and backward sway pg. 136

Side to side sway pg. 137

Warrior I pg. 138

Warrior II pg. 140

Lateral angle pg. 142

Chair pose pg. 144

Warrior III pg. 145

Tree pose pg. 147

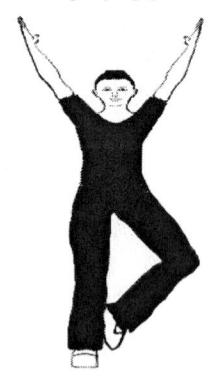

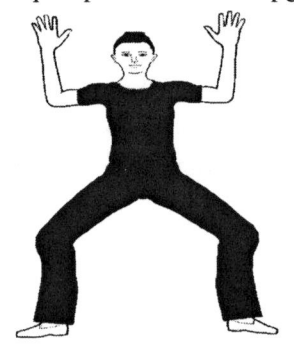

Victory squat pose/W stretch pg. 149

Dancer's pose pg. 151

Hamstring stretch 153

Seated half lotus pose pg. 155

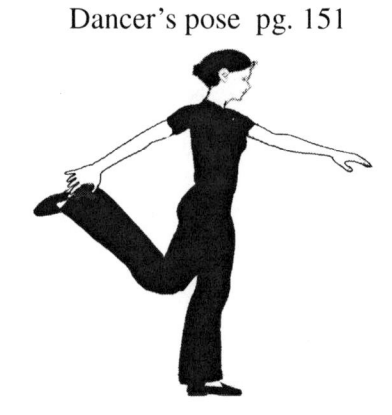

Seated spinal twist pg. 156

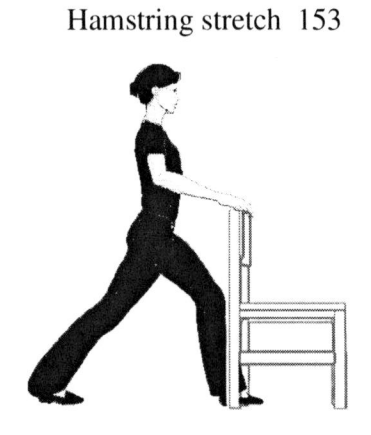

Knee to chest pg. 157

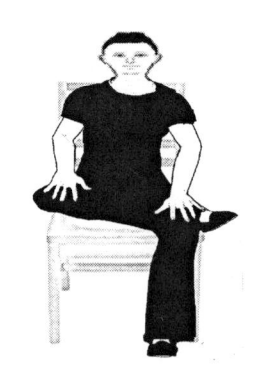

Ankle exercises pg. 158

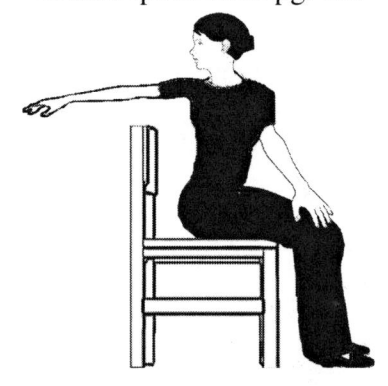

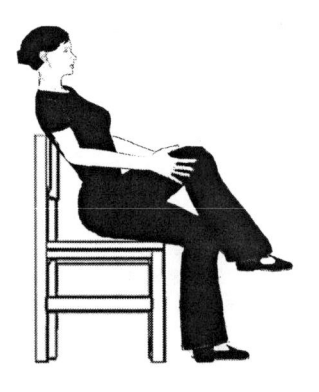

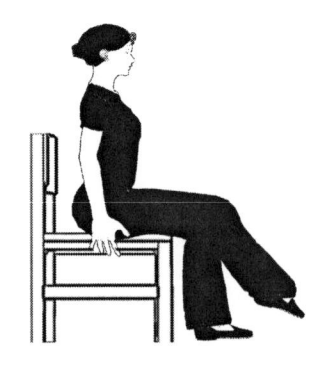

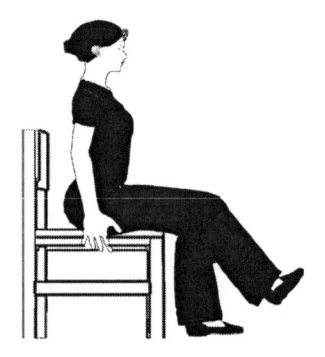

Floor Exercises

Pelvic tilts pg. 161

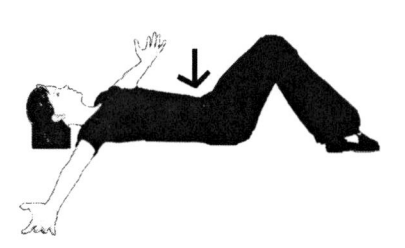

Knee to chest pg. 162

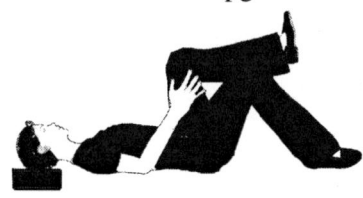

Bridge pg. 163

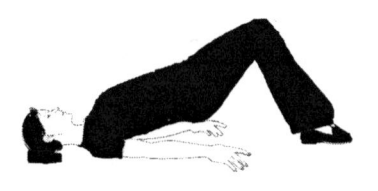

Overhead arm reach pg. 164

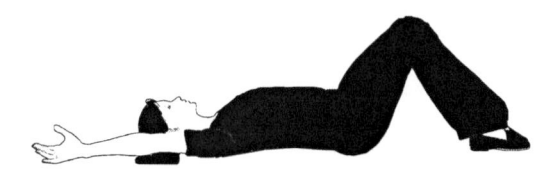

Double arm reach pg. 165

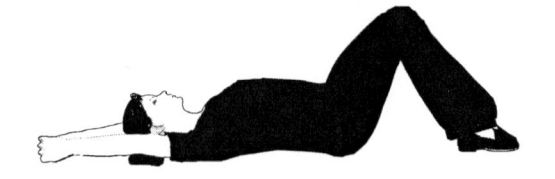

Leg lift pg. 166

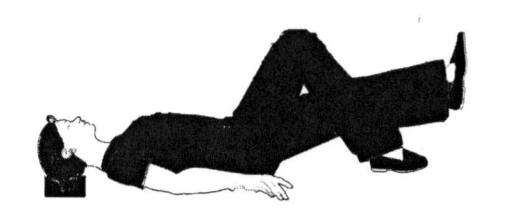

Opposite arm and leg reach pg. 167

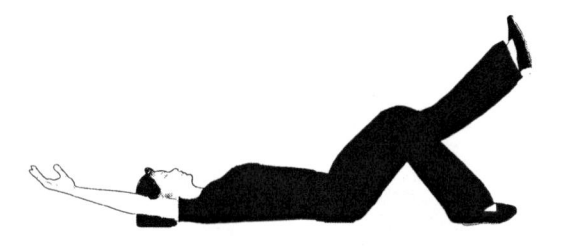

Hamstring stretch pg. 168

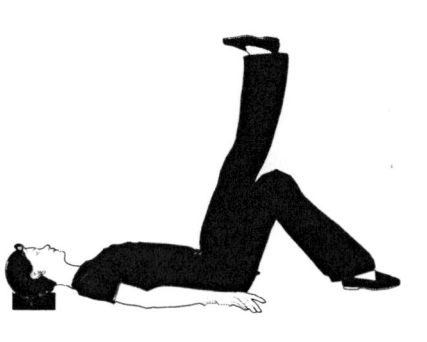

Spinal twist pg. 169

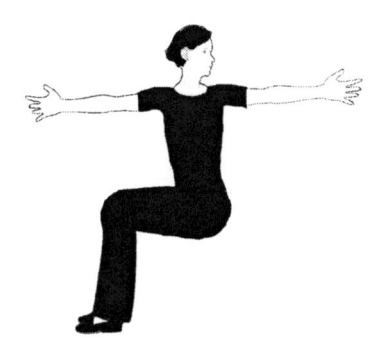

Bound angle pg. 170

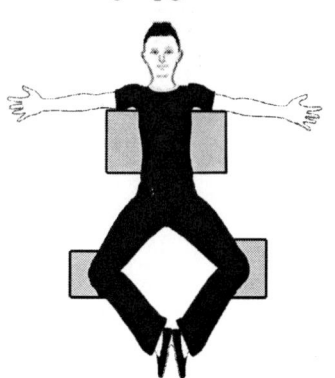

Tai Chi Reference Sheet

Refer to Chapter five for complete instructions. Most of the standing movements can also be done seated.

Press energy down pg. 174

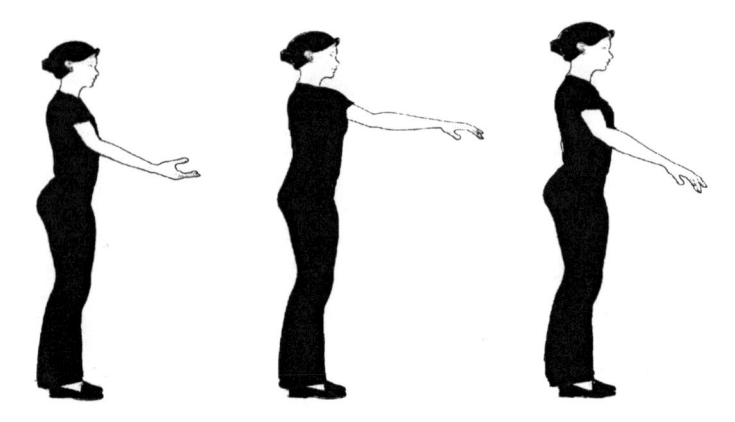

Spread the eagle's wings pg. 176

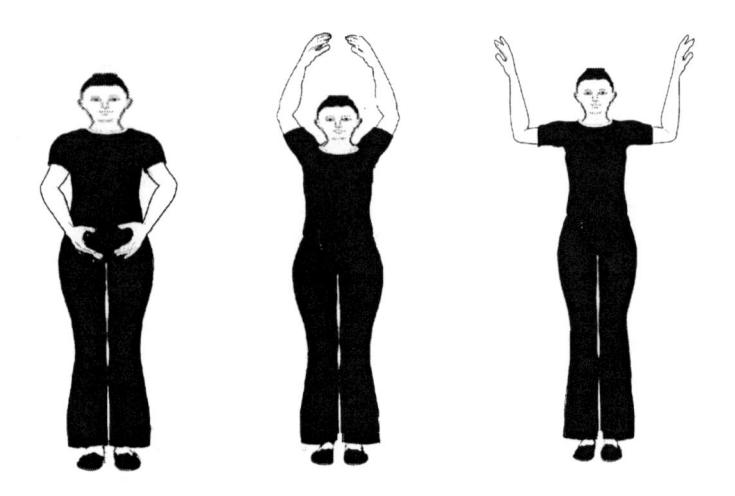

Gathering energy pg. 178

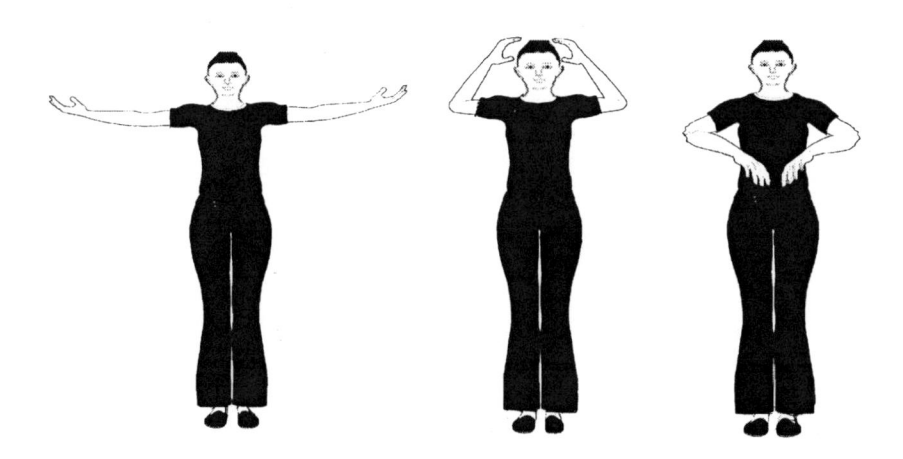

Waist twists pg. 180

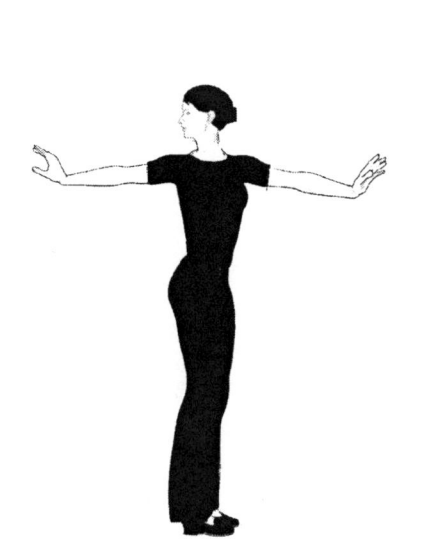

Side bends pg. 182

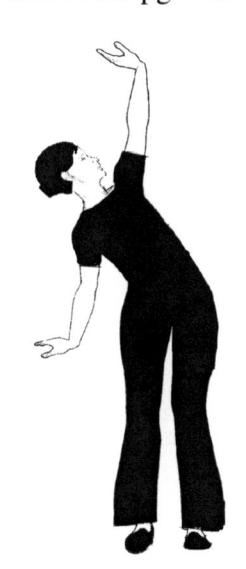

Tai chi walk pg 184

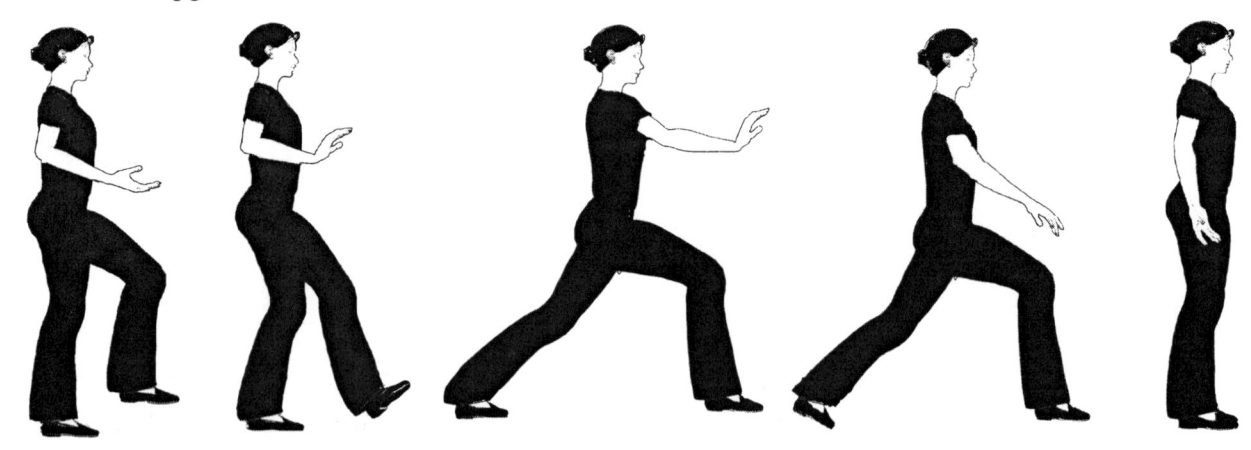

Chasing clouds pg 185

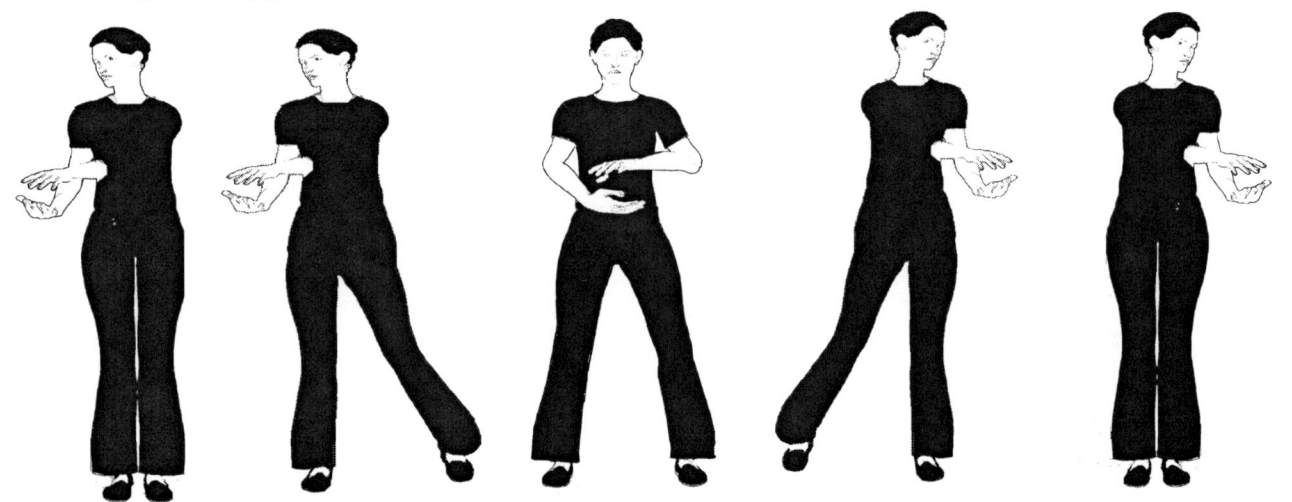

Tandem walking forward and backwards pg. 186

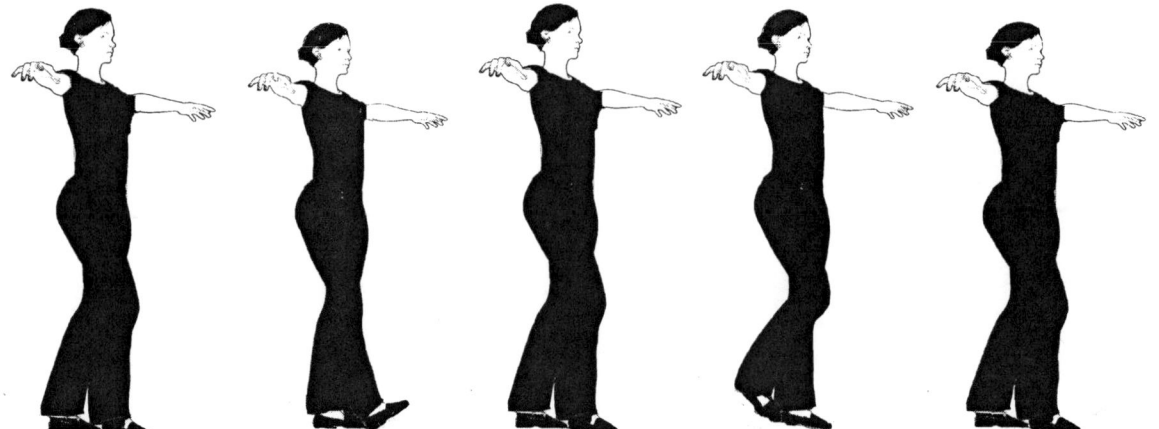

Diary for Stress Management/Meditation Exercises

Many of our clients have found it helpful to keep diaries or journals as part of their stress management program. Below is a sample page we use in our program. You can use one sheet for each time you practice or you may wish to write in a diary or journal.

Relaxation/Meditation Technique Used _____

Time of day you practiced _____

Length of time you practiced _____

How did you feel before your practice?

_____

_____

_____

_____

How did you feel after your practice?

_____

_____

_____

_____

List any experiences which you decided to respond to differently than you usually would.

_____

_____

_____

Resource Section

Biographies

Csuy, Jeanne PT, GCS, MS
 Jeanne is the Outreach Coordinator for Lee Parkinson Outreach Center in Fort Myers, Florida. Jeanne has been a physical therapist for over 40 years and has a physical therapy specialty certification in Geriatrics.

Van Hulsteyn, Peggy
 Peggy is the author of six books and a popular keynote speaker and has written about living with Parkinson's for *Yoga Journal*, American Parkinson Disease Association publications, and other travel and fitness magazines. Her articles on a wide range of additional subjects have appeared in the *Washington Post, Los Angeles Times, Miami Herald, Chicago Tribune, San Francisco Examiner,* and *USA Today,* as well as *Mademoiselle* and *Cosmopolitan* Magazines and periodicals published in Australia. Her work has been translated into Japanese, Spanish, Dutch, and Portuguese. She lives in Santa Fe, New Mexico with her physicist husband and two literary cats and is at work on a book titled Living Creatively with Parkinson's: A Guide to Empowerment.

Zylstra, Ann PT
 Ann Zylstra is the Supervisor of Evergreen's out patient rehabilitation services and the Booth Gardner Parkinson's Care Center's lead physical therapist. She has more than 21 years experience developing rehabilitation programs for patients with Parkinson's and other neurological problems that affect balance and gait. Ann is the co-president of the Washington Chapter of the APDA. Ann is also certified in vestibular rehabilitation.

Boylan Laura S., MD
 Laura is an Assistant Professor of Neurology at the New York University School of Medicine. A behavioral and cognitive neurologist, she completed medical school residency in neurology and a fellowship in affective disorders at Columbia University.
 Her research interests include aspects of mood disorders and emotional processing in neurobiological disorders including Parkinson's disease, epilepsy and primary mood disorders; she has numerous publications in these areas. Her clinical practice is at Bellevue Hospital in New York City

Helpful Organizations and Webpages

Information on Parkinson's Disease (Treatment, education, research and services)

The American Parkinson Disease Association, Inc.
135 Parkinson Avenue
Staten Island, NY 10305
1-800-223-2732
www.apdaparkinson.org

LSVT® (Lee Silverman Voice Treatment)
www.lsvt.org

The Michael J. Fox Foundation for Parkinson's Research
Church Street Station
P.O. Box 780
New York, NY 10008-0780
1-800-708-7644
www.michaeljfox.org

National Parkinson Foundation, Inc.
1501 N.W. 9th Avenue / Bob Hope Road
Miami, Florida 33136-1494
1-800-327-4545
www.parkinson.org

Northwest Parkinson's Disease Foundation
400 Mercer St., #401
Seattle, WA 98109
1-877-980.7500
www.nwpf.org

Parkinson's Disease Foundation Inc.
1359 Broadway, Suite 1509
New York, NY 10018
Phone: (212) 923-4700
www.pdf.org

Medline
Provides articles concerning research on Parkinson's disease
www.nlm.nih.gov/medlineplus/parkinsonsdisease.html

Information on fitness (Exercise, healthy lifestyle topics, finding a qualified instructor)

American College Of Sports Medicine
P.O. Box 1440
Indianapolis, IN 46206-1440
1-317- 637-9200
www.acsm.org

National Institute of Health
9000 Rockville Pike
Bethesda, Maryland 20892
1-301-496-4000
www.nih.gov

National Institute of Aging
Building 31, Room 5C27
31 Center Drive, MSC 2292
Bethesda, MD 20892
www.nih.gov/nia

Weil Lifestyle, LLC
Andrew Weil M.D.
www.drweil.com/

Information on yoga (Types of yoga, postures, books, videos, finding a qualified instructor)

Kripalu Center for Yoga and Health
PO Box 309
Stockbridge, MA 01262
1-866-200-5203
www.kripalu.org

National Yoga Alliance
1701 Clarendon Boulevard, Suite 110
Arlington, VA 22209
1-888-921-9642
www.yogaalliance.org

Yoga Journal
www.yogajournal.com

Information on stress management and meditation (Forms of meditation, techniques, videos)

Academy for Guided Imagery
30765 Pacific Coast Highway, Suite 369
Malibu, CA 90265
1-800-726-2070
www.academyforguidedimagery.com

Bernie Siegel/ECAP
522 Jackson Park Drive
Meadville, PA 16335
1-814-337-8192
www.ecap-online.org
www.berniesiegelmd.com/

Jon Kabat-Zin
Stress Reduction Tapes
P.O. Box 547
Lexington, MA 02420
www.mindfulnesstapes.com

Benson-Henry Institute for Mind Body Medicine
Massachusetts General Hospital
151 Merrimac Street
Boston, MA 02114
1-617-643-6090
http://www.massgeneral.org/bhi/

Thich Nhat Hahn
Plum Village
www.plumvillage.org

Umass Medical Center
The Center for Mindfulness in Medicine, Health Care, and Society
55 Lake Avenue
North Worcester, MA 01655
1-508-856-2656
www.umassmed.edu/cfm

Information on physical therapy

American Physical Therapy Association
1111 North Fairfax Street
Alexandria, VA 22314-1488
1-800-999-2782
www.apta.org

It is also helpful to check your local library for books, videos and CD's. They often have a wide selection of books on exercise, yoga, meditation and health management.

Index

A
Abdominal lean backs..................123
Aerobic exercise 77
Ankle exercises 158
Arm circles 71
Auditory system; and balance 129
Autogenic training 197

B
Balance; maintaining 129
Basic meditation exercise 195
Bent row 114
Biceps curl 119
Bicycle exercise 124
Body mechanics principals 16
Bound angle pose 170
Bridge pose 163

C
Cardiovascular system 80
Cat stretch 62
Chair pose 144
Chasing clouds 185
Chest fly 113
Chin tuck 57
Chest opener 63
Chest stretch 75

D
Dancer's pose 151
Deltoid raise 118
Diaphragmatic breathing 47

E
Effects of exercise on the heart 80
Effects of exercise on the respiratory system 82
Effects of meditation 195
Effects of stress on the body 189

F
Facial exercises..........................171
Falls; causes of..........................128
Fight or flight syndrome..............191
Flexibility...................................132
Freezing; tips to get moving..........79

G
Gathering energy........................178
Getting in and out of bed..............29
Getting in and out of a car............25
Getting in and out of a chair.........21
Getting up and down from the floor....42
Grooming tips..............................34
Guided imagery.........................199

H
Hamstring stretch standing..........153
Hamstring stretch seated.............154
Hamstring stretch on floor...........168
Head rotations/stretch...................55
Heel curls....................................90
Heel lifts......................................66
Heel taps.....................................93
Heel raises.................................108
Hip hinge.....................................18
Hip stretch.................................155
Housework and posture................37

K
Knee lifts.....................................89
Knee to chest stretch seated.......157
Knee to chest stretch on floor.....162

231

L
Lateral angle pose..................................142
Lateral raise..116
Leg crossover......................................106
Leg extension......................................100
Leg lift standing..................................102
Leg lift on floor...................................166
Lifting correctly....................................39

M
Making exercise part of your day...........11
Marching in place..................................85
Meditation..195
Meditation diary..................................225
Military press......................................117
Mindfulness meditation.......................202
Mountain pose.....................................135
Music for aerobics.................................79

N
Neck rolls/stretch..................................52
Nervous system..................................190

O
Opposite arm to leg reach on floor.......167
Overhead double arm reach on floor...165
Overhead single arm reach on floor....164
Overhead stretch...................................74

P
Pelvic tilt on floor................................151
Pressing energy down.........................174
Putting on shoes...................................36

Q
Quadriceps stretch...............................150

R
Rating of perceived exertion..................78
Reference sheet for aerobic exercises...211
Reference sheet for strength training exercises..214
Reference sheet for yoga postures......219
Reference sheet for tai chi exercises...222
Reference sheet for warm-up exercises..........209
Reverse wrist curls...............................122

S
Sample aerobic routines........................94
Sample exercise routines.....................206
Shoulder rolls..58
Side bend/stretch..................................67
Side bend; with weights......................126
Side leg lift..102
Side toe taps...91
Sitting correctly.....................................19
Spinal twist/stretch; warm-up...............59
Spinal twist; yoga................................156
Spinal twist on floor............................169
Spreading the eagle's wings................176
Squats; warm up...................................72
Squats; strength training......................98
Standing correctly.................................26
Stepping side to side.............................87
Straight leg kicks...................................86
Strength training...................................97
Stress..189
Stress and Parkinson's disease............194
Stretching tips.....................................132
Swaying forward and back..................136
Swaying side to side............................137

232

T

Tai chi	173
Tai chi side bends	182
Tai chi walk	184
Talk test	78
Tandem walking	186
Ten rep max	97
Tree pose	147
Triceps kickback	120
Toe lifts	65

V

Victory squat pose	149
Visual system; and balance	129
Voice projection exercises	172

W

Waists twists	180
Walking correctly	27
Wall pushups	112
Wall slides	99
Warrior I pose	138
Warrior II pose	140
Warrior III pose	145
Web pages; helpful	227
Workout log; aerobic	212
Workout log; strength training	217
Wrist curls	121

Y

Yoga	128

For more information on our other products and workshops

Visit us at:

Living Well Yoga and Fitness
www.lwyf.org